HEMOSTASIS RESEARCH

CLOTTING DISORDERS

SYMPTOMS, DIAGNOSIS AND MANAGEMENT

HEMOSTASIS RESEARCH

Additional books in this series can be found on Nova's website under the Series tab.

Additional e-books in this series can be found on Nova's website under the e-book tab.

HEMOSTASIS RESEARCH

CLOTTING DISORDERS

SYMPTOMS, DIAGNOSIS AND MANAGEMENT

JEFFREY L. WILSON
EDITOR

NOVA BIOMEDICAL
New York

Additional color graphics may be available in the e-book version of this book.

Library of Congress Cataloging-in-Publication Data

ISBN: 978-1-63482-830-7
Library of Congress Control Number: 2015939094

Published by Nova Science Publishers, Inc. † New York

Contents

Preface

Coagulopathy (also called clotting disorder and bleeding disorder) is a condition in which the blood's ability to clot (coagulate) is impaired. Acquired hemophilia is a rare disorder characterized by spontaneous bleeding in a patient with no previous personal or family hemorrhagic history. The first chapter explores the challenges associated with this disease, its unfamiliarity often causing a delay in diagnosis and therapeutic approaches. The second chapter focuses on lower gastrointestinal bleeding (LGIB) in children, describing the epidemiology, etiology and clinical management. The third chapter reviews the pathogenesis, risk factors and treatment strategies of coagulopathy in patients with craniocerebral injury. The next article examines Vitamin B12 with its four cobalamin vitamers, which often play a role in coagulation. The next chapter starts with a description of the methodology of viscoelastic hemostatic assay, followed by a review of literature on the utilization of thrombelastography (TEG) or rotational thromboelastometry (ROTEM). Finally, the role of TEG and ROTEM to monitor or guide prophylaxis/treatment of thromboembolic events and the limitations of using them to detect hypercoagulability and identify patients with increased risks for thromboembolic complications are discussed. The final chapter of this book focuses on the use of fresh frozen plasma (FFP) in patients who are not actively bleeding, critically questions these assumptions in the context of pre-procedural administration of FFP, and also examines why carrying out high quality trails in this area has been so problematic.

Chapter 1 – Acquired hemophilia is a disorder difficult to diagnose, with little prevalence, aged biphasic appearance and predominance of the female sex at early ages. Its diagnosis is often difficult, however, in recent years, everyone was worried about having adequate laboratory techniques that meet the criteria of standardization to reduce the possibility of false positive or negative. In 40-50% of cases there is usually an underlying cause that explains the development of the disease, however, in the rest of the population there is not an underlying cause. This is quite important to identified, because removing or handling the trigger is essential to achieve an eradication of the inhibitor and control the disease. Where it is not possible to identify the trigger, the treatment approach is based on making use of immunosuppressive drugs (steroids, alkylating cytostatic agents, imidazole derivative of 6-mercaptopurine drugs, among others) based on different international protocols.

Chapter 2 – Gastrointestinal bleeding (GIB) is a relatively common event in the pediatric population, it can potentially occur anywhere in the enteric canal which is highly vascularised. It is important to investigate appropriately every child presenting with GIB, keeping in mind that this phenomenon can be the presenting sign for heterogeneous pathologies with different severity, ranging from benign conditions that require little if any intervention to severe diseases including surgical emergencies, inflammatory bowel disease (IBD) and clotting disorders. The term GIB includes both upper gastrointestinal bleeding (UGIB) and lower gastrointestinal bleeding (LGIB). The former refers to bleeding that originates proximal to the ligament of Treitz, the latter bleeding distal to the ligament of Treitz. The present review chapter focuses on LGIB in children, describing epidemiology, etiology according to children's age and proposes a practical algorithm for clinical management. LGIB represents 0.3% of the referrals to a Pediatric Emergency Department and is usually a benign condition which resolves spontaneously in 80% of cases. However, in approximately 20% of cases it may be the sign of severe disease or potentially life threatening conditions. The etiology of LGIB in pediatric age varies significantly according to the child's age. For example, in neonatal age frequent causes are represented by swallowed maternal blood and surgical emergencies such as necrotizing enterocolitis, malrotation with midgut volvulus and hirschsprung's disease. In infancy (age range 1 month-2 years), the causes are heterogenous ranging from anorectal fissures and allergic proctitis to more severe diseases such as hemolytic uremic syndrome, henoch-schönlein purpura and surgical conditions including intussusception and meckel's diverticulum. In pre-school children (age range 2-5 years) infectious diarrhoea, gastrointestinal polyps and polyposis syndromes are the most common causes of LGIB. In school-aged children and adolescents, the spectrum of disorders with LGIB is similar to that of preschool children, with the exception that IBD often occurs in this age range. Besides the above described diseases which are typical of children in specific age ranges, several clotting disorders may be responsible of LGIB across all pediatric ages.

In fact, coagulopathies (either congenital or acquired) and thrombocytopenias (either idiopathic or secondary), besides presenting more commonly with epistaxis, hematoma's and hemathrosis may more rarely present with acute gastrointestinal bleeding. In the clinical management of LGIB a two-step approach can be proposed. The first step is to assess the general well-being of the patient, and to treat or prevent hemodynamic instability. After assessment of hemodynamic stability and stabilisation of critical patients the second step is to distinguish UGIB from LGIB and if possible to identify the site of GIB. A thorough history, and an accurate physical examination followed by laboratory and imaging tests represent the cornerstone of LGIB work-up.

Chapter 3 – Head trauma, a common neurosurgical emergency, is associated with high mortality and morbidity rates. Coagulation disorders, which may be present in head trauma, are associated with worse outcome and increased mortality. There are two major groups of coagulation disorders with essential impact on the outcome after head trauma, which are anticoagulant and antiplatelet therapy and coagulopathy following traumatic brain injury. The first type, with increased occurrence, is caused by the increased use of anticoagulant and antiplatelet treatment in population for cardiovascular diseases. The second type, which may be present in approximately 30-40 % of traumatic brain injury patients, is coagulation disorder following traumatic brain injury. It is characterised by the release of tissue factor and activation of pro-coagulant factors, resulting in complex thrombin formation and conversion of fibrinogen to fibrin. Both types of coagulopathy increase the risk of poor outcome and death among patients with brain trauma.

If the intracranial pressure increases and incranial hypertension occurs, emergency neurosurgical intervention is necessary. Coagulation disorder is a relative contraindication for surgery. On the other hand, surgery leads to consumption of pro-coagulant factors, which may aggravate pre-existing coagulopathy.

Chapter 4 – *Background:* Cobalamin is the hydrophilic vitamin B_{12} of a complicated structure with a central cobalt ion for normal erythropoiesis and nerve function. Vitamin B_{12} can clinically be given as 1000-1500 μg injections. Therefore, this work quantified the changed thrombin generation by altered matrix (AM) thru an increase of plasmatic vitamin B_{12} concentration.

Material and Methods: 40 μl platelet poor citrated plasma of 12 healthy donors were supplemented either with 0-610 μg/l hydroxocobalamin acetate or with 0-610 μg/l cyanocobalamine by repetitive 1+1 dilution on the polystyrene microtiter plate (Brand®781600). The RECA was performed with 10 or 20 min (37°C) coagulation reaction time. The approx. SC200 or approx. IC50 was determined for each individual plasma.

Results and Discussion: The approx. SC200 on AM-coagulation was 19±14 μg/l (MV±1SD) hydroxocobalamin acetate in 5 of 6 plasmas; one plasma had an approx. IC50 of 8 μg/l. Cyanocobalamin had an approx. SC200 of 101±130 μg/l in 3 of 6 plasmas and an approx. IC50 of 13±14 μg/l in 3 of 6 samples. This means that there are hemostasis differences between hydroxocobalamin acetate and cyanocobalamin. Hydroxocobalamin acetate triggers intrinsic coagulation much more than cyanocobalamin. This might be due to the acetate part of the hydroxocobalamin drug. It could be of pharmacologic interest to substitute acetate in hydroxocobalamin by HCl.

Chapter 5 – Practice guidelines continue to give somewhat conflicting advice regarding indications for Fresh Frozen Plasma (FFP) transfusion and it is therefore not surprising that repeatedly worldwide, audits of FFP usage demonstrate abundant inappropriate transfusion. Nearly half of all FFP transfusions are given prophylactically in order to correct prolonged prothrombin time (PT) and/or international normalized ratio (INR) prior to an invasive or operative procedure in the absence of bleeding. However, the evidence supporting this practice is very poor and will be reviewed in this chapter. Meta-analyses fail to demonstrate that elevated PT and/or INR predict(s) bleeding across a wide range of specialities. Global assays of hemostasis such as viscoelastography may be more useful in predicting bleeding risk but large-scale outcome studies are required. Studies in different patient populations show that coagulation factor levels are generally well above the threshold for adequate hemostasis (30%) until the INR exceeds 2.0 x control. In addition, FFP does not reliably correct INR values ≤ 1.8 x control unless given in volumes much larger than conventional doses. Specific clinical scenarios where prophylactic FFP transfusions often occur include patients with liver disease, procedures in critical care, cardiac and liver surgery and warfarin reversal. There is little evidence to support plasma transfusion in any of these situations and the risks of transfusion are not insignificant, including transfusion related acute lung injury (TRALI), transfusion associated circulatory overload (TACO), delays in procedures and increased cost. Clinical trials looking at bleeding risks with or without plasma transfusion have been difficult to carry out and the challenges encountered will be reviewed in this chapter. Deeply-engrained personal beliefs and lack of evidence continue to fuel prophylactic FFP transfusion by clinicians; the call for clinical trials has never been greater.

In: Clotting Disorders
Editor: Jeffrey L. Wilson

ISBN: 978-1-63482-830-7

Chapter 1

Acquired Hemophilia

Nicolas Coronel–Restrepo [1], MD, Maria Fernanda Alvarez–Barreneche [2], MD, and Kenny Galvez–Cardenas [3], MD

[1]Resident of Internal Medicine, CES University, Medellín, Colombia
[2]Resident of Internal Medicine, Pontificia Bolivariana University, Medellín, Colombia
[3]Specialist in Hematology, Hospital Pablo Tobon Uribe, Medellin, Colombia

Abstract

Acquired hemophilia is a disorder difficult to diagnose, with little prevalence, aged biphasic appearance and predominance of the female sex at early ages. Its diagnosis is often difficult, however, in recent years, everyone was worried about having adequate laboratory techniques that meet the criteria of standardization to reduce the possibility of false positive or negative. In 40-50% of cases there is usually an underlying cause that explains the development of the disease, however, in the rest of the population there is not an underlying cause. This is quite important to identified, because removing or handling the trigger is essential to achieve an eradication of the inhibitor and control the disease. Where it is not possible to identify the trigger, the treatment approach is based on making use of immunosuppressive drugs (steroids, alkylating cytostatic agents, imidazole derivative of 6-mercaptopurine drugs, among others) based on different international protocols.

Introduction

Acquired hemophilia is a rare disorder characterized by spontaneous bleeding in a patient with no previous personal or family hemorrhagic history. It is usually associated with the presence of circulating autoantibodies that inhibit the activity of a particular coagulation factor. More frequently against factor (F) VIII, von Willebrand factor (VWF) and less frequently against factors V, IX, XI and XIII. In most cases, bleeding episodes are spontaneous and severe at presentation.

The treatment has been extrapolated from the management of congenital hemophilia A with inhibitors. To date there are few studies that provide strong recommendations for the management of these patients, including the use of bypassing agents as first-line therapy; immunosuppressive therapy for the eradication of the inhibitor and resolution of the etiologic factor.

The disease is a clinical challenge and its unfamiliarity makes a delay in diagnosis and therapeutic approach. This delay will have a negative impact on rates of bleeding and thus mortality.

1. Definition

When we refer to Acquired hemophilia, we are talking about a rare disorder characterized by spontaneous bleeding without personal or family history of bleeding. It is characterized by autoantibodies that inhibit the activity of a particular factor. More often against FVIII, VWF, less frequently against FV, FIX, FXI and FXIII. Only a few isolated reports against fibrinogen, FVII and FX are known [1]. It must be distinguished from congenital hemophilia, which is an inherited disorder caused by mutations in the FVIII gene that presents at a young age and is characterized by a distinct bleeding phenotype. [2]

Epidemiology

This disease is a clinical challenge. Currently the worldwide data about this disease are very few. The presence of severe bleeding, concomitant diseases, subestimation of symptoms, the delay in diagnostic and therapeutic approach, are characteristics that make this disease with a high mortality rate [3]. As a rare disease, the information we have about this entity is thanks to records and demographic characterizations carried out mainly in Australia [4], Wales [5] and United Kingdom [6], so far there is no records in Latin America. In 1981, with the analysis of doctors Green and Lechner [7], the first data about the entity were obtained (Table 1).

Acquired inhibitors against FVIII occur rarely in the non-haemophilic population, with a reported incidence of approximately one case per million/year [5] and the incidence increases with age, being a very uncommon disease in children. The incidence in children younger than 16 years has been estimated to be 0.045 per million/year compared with 14.7 per million/year in the elderly aged older than 85 years, although epidemiologic data are likely to be underestimated in elderly patients [6]. The incidence in men and women is similar except in the age range 20 to 40 years, when the effect of pregnancy results in a preponderance in women [8]. In approximately 50% of cases, FVIII autoantibodies occur in patients lacking any relevant concomitant disease, while the remaining cases may be associated with postpartum period, autoimmune diseases, underlying hematologic or solid cancers, infections, or use of medications [9].

To date, the largest prospective database data that exist is the pan-European registration EACH2 (European Acquired Haemophilia Registry) [10]. These study included 117 centers in 13 different European countries and in five countries including 43 different centers in Finland, Greece, Hungary, Italy and Portugal the authorities did not allow the analysis of data from patients who died, a situation that could affect the final results. One interesting fact of this record was that a central laboratory for analysis of the samples was not used and allowed each center to make individually analyzing of the blood samples, being the reflection of interlaboratory variability in the real world. According to EACH2 data, acquired hemophilia has a biphasic distribution between 20 to 37 years (mean age: 33.9 years) and between 40 and 90 years (mean age: 73.9 years). The prospective UK study [6], showed a median age of diagnosed patients of 78 years. More than 80% of patients being 65 years or older.

Table 1. Comparison of the results of different cohorts

Study	Year of the study	Number of patients in the study	Age of occurrence of the disease	Gender predilection	Incidence of disease	Underlying disorder [n (%)]	Drugs associated with the presence of inhibitors	No etiologic factor associated [n (%)]	Main site bleeding
Green and Lechner [7]	1981	Questionnaire given to 215 patients with FVIII inhibitors	Mostly > 50 years old	No difference by gender predilection. Male sex 53%	ND	Malignancy (Any type): 12 (6.4) Autoimmune disorder: 32 (17.0) Postpartum: 13 (7.0) Infections: ND Dermatological conditions: 8 (4.3) Drug induced: 10 (5.3) Others: 21 (16.5)	In several there was an association with allergy to penicillin,	82 (43.6%)	Major bleeding was observed in 87% of patients, and in 22%, death was attributed either directly or indirectly to the presence of the inhibitor.
Australia, Tay L, et al., [4]	1997 – 2008	25 patients retrospectively over 12 years	Median age of 78 years	Equivalent sex ratio (12 males versus 13 females)	1.20 cases per million/year	Advanced age and lack of treatment were predictive of poor survival outcomes. The very elderly (>75 years of age) may warrant a different treatment modality such as rituximab, which is potentially more tolerable and efficacious.	ND	ND	ND

Study	Year of the study	Number of patients in the study	Age of occurrence of the disease	Gender predilection	Incidence of disease	Underlying disorder [n (%)]	Drugs associated with the presence of inhibitors	No etiologic factor associated [n (%)]	Main site bleeding
Wales, Collins P et al., [5]	1996 – 2002	Report on a consecutive, unselected cohort of all patients in south and west Wales. There were 18 patients	Median age of 70 years	12 males versus 6 females	1.34 per million/year	Less likely to have an underlying diagnosis (27%)	ND	95 (63.3%)	The bleeding phenotype was less severe, with only 27% having life or limb threatening bleeds and 41% required no haemostatic treatment.
United Kingdom, Collins PW et al., [6]	2001 – 2003	Consecutive cohort of patients, unbiased by referral or reporting practice. A total of 172 patients	Median age of 78 years. The cohort was significantly older than previously reported series	Of the 122 patients whose sex was reported, just under half (43%) were men although in the age group 21 to 40 years, all 4 patients were women	1.5 cases per million/year, which increased with age, as estimated to be 0.045 per million/year in children under 16 years and 14.7 per million/ year in the elderly aged over 85 years	Malignancy (Any type): 22 (14.7) Autoimmune disorder: 25 (16.7) Postpartum: 3 (2.0) Infections: ND Dermatological conditions: 5 (3.3) Drug induced: ND Others: ND	ND	An underlying diagnosis was found in all of the 5 patients under age 40 years, 55% of those between 40 and 59 years, 42% of those between	Bleeding manifestations and underlying diseases were similar. Many patents had more than one type of bleeding

Table 1. (Continued)

Study	Year of the study	Number of patients in the study	Age of occurrence of the disease	Gender predilection	Incidence of disease	Underlying disorder [n (%)]	Drugs associated with the presence of inhibitors	No etiologic factor associated [n (%)]	Main site bleeding
								60 and 79 years, and 23% of those aged 80 or over	
EACH2, Knoebl P et al., [8]	2003 – 2008	117 centers in 13 different European countries, total 501 patients were included (266 men and 235 women)	Biphasic distribution between 20 to 37 years (mean age: 33.9 years) and the other between 40 and 90 years (mean age: 73.9 years).	No gender variation in the older group. In the younger age group, a higher incidence in women. Fifty-seven per cent of the non-pregnancy-related cases were male.	ND	Malignancy (Any type): 59 (11.9%) Autoimmune disorder: 67 (13.4) Postpartum: 42 (8.4) Infections: 19 (3.8) Dermatological conditions: 7 (1.4) Drug induced: 17 (3.4) Others: 58 (11.6)	Exposure to beta-lactam antibiotics (23.5%), clopidogrel (17.6%), other non – beta-lactamic antibiotics , transfusion and NSAIDs (11.8%) were the most involved in the development of the disease	260 (51.9%)	Unusual bleeding in CNS and hemarthrosis. Retroperitoneal bleeding and skeletal muscle were characteristic of gravity level requiring transfusion support. 89% of patients had some kind of manifestation of bleeding that preceded the diagnosis. After bleeding the

Study	Year of the study	Number of patients in the study	Age of occurrence of the disease	Gender predilection	Incidence of disease	Underlying disorder [n (%)]	Drugs associated with the presence of inhibitors	No etiologic factor associated [n (%)]	Main site bleeding
									diagnosis had an average delay of three days.
Metanalysis Delgado et al., [23]	1985-2002	20 surveys retrospective and prospective, 249 patients (range 5–34 patients per article). Fifteen patients were lost to follow-up and excluded from analysis.	64 years (range 8–93 years), with a typical bimodal distribution	55% females 45% males	ND	Related conditions, Malignancy 43 (18), post partum 34 (15), autoimmune disorders 22 (9), others or unidentified 135 (58)	ND	Others or unidentified 135 (58)	ND

ND: no data

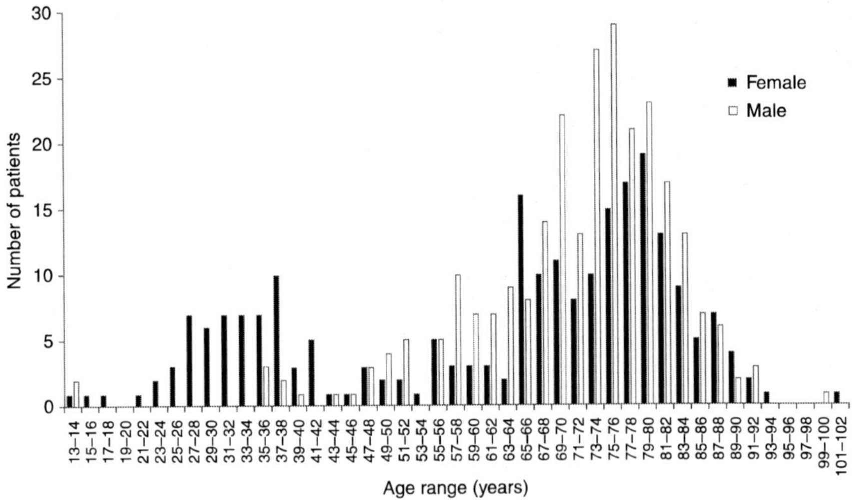

Figure 1. Age distribution of patients with Acquired hemophilia. Reprinted with the permission of the author from EACH2.

2. Pathophysiological Concepts

It is unknown what there are predisposing factors for the disease development [1, 8, 9]. It is likely that a mixture of genetic factors like alterations in allelic HLA II, specially specific single nucleotide polymorphisms (SNPs) of the CTLA-4 lymphocyte, in the midst of an environment that predisposes the loss of immune tolerance.

FVIII is a protein with a molecular weight of 265Kd whose amino acid sequences are grouped into six domains. Thus, A1, A2 and B domains are grouped on the heavy chain while A3, C1 and C2 domains are in the light chain [11]. Usually, the autoantibodies are directed against a single domain unlike alloantibodies that would be directed against one or more domains; this phenomenon probably explains the difference in clinical bleeding phenotypes between, acquired hemophilia and the development of alloantibodies associated with the use of exogenous factors, such as recombinant factor VIIa (rFVIIa) and activated prothrombin complex concentrate (FEIBA). Usually these inhibitors are directed against the A2 and A3 domains (inhibits binding to FIXa) and C2 (inhibits vWF binding, FXa and FIXa). These antibodies are usually immunoglobulin (Ig) G polyclonal IgG1 and IgG4 subtypes [3], with occasional reports of IgA or IgM monoclonal nature [11]; apparently dependent on the type of stimulation do CD4 T lymphocyte. When there is a predominance of Th1 response, the prevailing immunoglobulin subtypes are IgG1 and IgG2. Conversely, when the response is Th2 mediated the inhibitory response will be IgG4. This is clinically important, because the antibodies developed by Th1 satisfactorily respond to therapeutic measures unlike Th2 responses wich have more intensive and more severe inhibitory response and higher serum levels [3].

3. Clinical Aspects

The most striking difference between auto- and alloantibodies is their FVIII inactivation pattern. It has been described two types of responses: type 1 (or first order kinetics) which refers to the typical behavior of alloantibodies which are capable of completely inactivate FVIII if inhibitor is present in excess, usually in this type of inhibition the levels of FVIII are related with the severity of bleeding. In the other hand, type 2 (or 2 order kinetics) is not a linear response as type 1, this is characterized by a rapid initial inactivation, followed by a slow phase; there is not a complete inhibition of FVIII even with very high concentrations of the inhibitor (Figure 2) [12]. Thus, the Bethesda assay, which quantifies the in vitro inhibitor titre, may underestimate the in vivo inhibitor potency, due to non-linear reaction kinetics [13]. Consequently, inhibitor titres or residual FVIII activity do not correlate closely with the bleeding phenotype and severe bleeding may occur even in the presence of relatively high (up to 10-20% of normal) FVIII levels. It is likely that the patient's age and comorbidities are those that influence the clinical phenotype.

The bleeding pattern of AHA is rather different from that of congenital haemophilia A. From the clinical standpoint, the bleeding pattern of acquired hemophilia is often spontaneous or traumatic, typically with compromised skin, muscle, soft tissue and mucocutaneus (e.g. epistaxis, gastrointestinal and urological bleeds) [6] whereas haemarthroses, a typical feature of congenital FVIII deficiency, are uncommon [8,10].

Severe or life-threatening bleeds, which involve most frequently the gastrointestinal tract and the retroperitoneal space, occur in 70-90% of patients, being fatal in 5-10% of cases [14]. The manifestations of severe bleeding are often associated with neoplastic diseases while those with no serious bleeding are associated with autoimmune diseases, according to EACH2.

As we already mentioned, not only the disease itself, some concomitant diseases, including cancers, autoimmune diseases, predispose the patient for a poor outcome. Clinical conditions associated with AHA include solid tumours and lymphoproliferative malignancies [15–19], autoimmune disorders (systemic lupus erythematosus, rheumatoid arthritis, Sjogren syndrome or thyroid disorders) [20–24], skin diseases (pemphigus and epidermolysis bullosa), drugs (penicillin and interferon) and infections (hepatitis B and C viruses) [25–29].

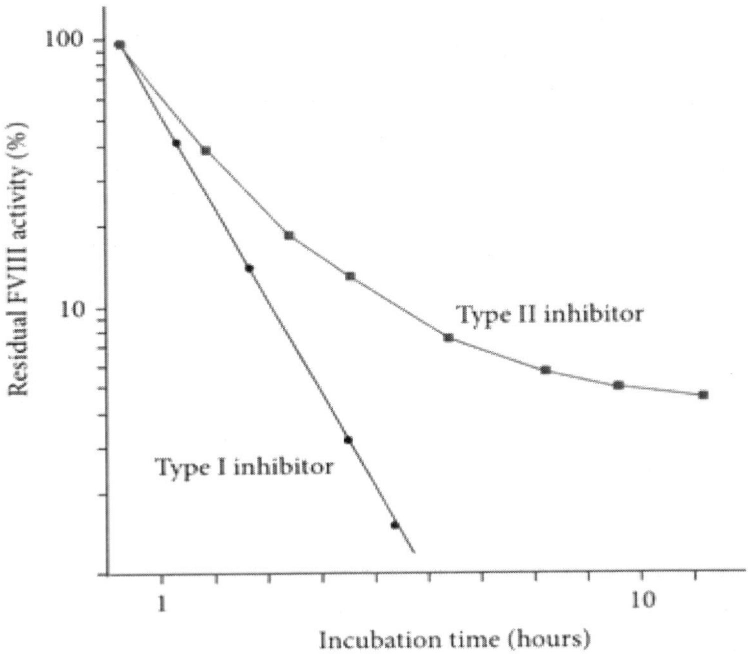

Figure 2. Kinetics of the inhibitors.

In the younger group the increase in incidence is possibly a reflection of the greater number of cases in women in pregnancy and especially the puerperium, as we already mentioned above [30,31]. The incidence may be variable, ranging from 2 to 21%. The EACH2 record showed that of 42 total pregnant women, 31 (74%) had acquired hemophilia in the first pregnancy and subsequent pregnancies curiously decreased the incidence (17%, 5%, 5% in the first, second and third pregnancy respectively). The mortality of acquired hemophilia in pregnancy is low (0 to 6%), possibly related to the low power and low levels of inhibitors in blood; however, the risk of bleeding is imminent, as it is the possibility of transplacental passage of autoantibodies [32].

Inhibitors usually appear 1-4 months after birth with an average of 77 days according to the registry EACH2. Sometimes they appear during labour, leading to severe blood loss [30]. It is important to keep in mind, that up to 60% of patients do not have a clear trigger factor explaining the development of the disease. These idiopathic form of the disease have been associated with aging and it has been concluded that it is possible that the probability of having a comorbidity associated with acquired hemophilia is inversely related to age [1].

4. Diagnostic Approach

It is likely, as demonstrated by Doctor Melissa Arbuckle in 2003 in patients with lupus [33], that the presence of autoantibodies (autoimmunity) may precede by many years the development of overt disease (autoimmunity manifests); so, you may encounter patients with prolonged aPTT (activated thromboplastin time) even without the presence of major bleeding and this would it be the only manifestation of acquired hemophilia. In order, to understand the different diagnostic tests that exist for addressing acquired hemophilia is important to understand the interaction between autoantibodies and alloantibodies to FVIII, as was exposed before (type 1 and 2 kinetics), in the type 2 kinetics there is no correlation between the FVIII and bleeding, under this premise, it is recommended that the antibodies and FVIII must be measured simultaneously in the plasma of patients [12].

To date there are not epidemiological studies of high power to give strong recommendations regarding the diagnosis and therapeutic approach, the evidence that is supported is based on large cohorts as EACH2, as we already mentioned. They all agree that the ideal way for the diagnosis of coagulation inhibitors is by studying mixtures 1: 1 [34–36]. is important to note that only requires 30 to 40% of the factor to normalize the aPTT. Once the study of mixtures has been made, those aPTT that corrects will be secondary to deficiency of factors while those who do not is due to the presence of an inhibitor. To analyze mixtures tests, it is important to understand that there are two types of inhibitors; one that are specific and those others who are not (global), specific antibodies are immunoglobulins that are usually directed against a specific coagulation factor or are directed against membrane phospholipids proteins such as lupus anticoagulant, hence the importance that when the test mixtures were made also a phospholipid sensitive test is performed, type time Russell viper venom, to rule out or confirm an associated antiphospholipid syndrome. The lupus anticoagulant may be normal in the presence of FVIII inhibitor, but can also falsely reduce levels of FVIII and simulate an acquired hemophilia. Furthermore global antibodies partially correct and are characterized to affect more than one part of the coagulation process, some examples of these kind of inhibitors are degradation products of fibrinogen, the monoclonal paraprotein and exposure to heparin [37]. Specific inhibitors in turn, may be neutralizing, when they directly inhibit factor activity, usually they are time - temperature dependent and are characterized by altering *in vitro* coagulation tests (example; aFVIII, aFIX, aFXI, aFXII, aFVII, aFX, aFV, aFII, aFIIa, aFVW), Unlike nonneutralizing inhibitor they do not inhibit the function of the factor and its pathophysiological mechanism is mediated by increasing the clearance of the same. Usually most of the inhibitors are fast acting, unlike those affecting FVIII and 15% of lupus anticoagulants that are slow acting. Factor VIII is labile compared with others and as we had already exposed the inhibitory capacity of antibodies is dependent on temperature and time, this explains the reason why 1: 1 mix required incubation at 37 Celsius for 2 hours with the aim to avoid false negative [37,38]. One aspect that has generated controversy and for which there is no international consensus, is how much is necessary to correct the aPTT to define that there is deficit of coagulation factors [12], the most accepted value is a percentage of correction more than 50% of aPTT, otherwise consider the presence of inhibitor [39], however, this is a very arbitrary definition, since the results and therefore the definition varies according to the protocols used in different laboratories, so it is proposed that if after mixing test, the upper limit of laboratory reference value is reached more than 5 seconds must consider the probability of correctness and therefore correction of factor deficit [12,40]. There are other methods for assessing the degree of correction as the Rosner index that quantifies the amount of correction of the aPTT patient with normal plasma, is considered correct if the Rosner index <15. Chang percentage is another formula that incorporates the degree of correction with respect to the prolongation of aPTT with a correction point of cut of 50%. Once it has been demonstrated the presence of inhibitors for the study of blends, the next step is to perform a measurement of the activity of FVIII and inhibitors; FVIII activity is measured with chromogenic studies and antibody titers are determined by Bethesda Test incorporated in 1975. It is important to be clear that this test was developed with the aim of determining alloantibodies (antibodies with first order kinetics or type 1), hence the interpretation of autoantibodies (Type 2) can be difficult in some circumstances [2]. The test is unique to quantify the antibody inhibitory activity (neutralizing) after incubation of normal plasma with various dilutions of patient plasma, and is then evaluated, the ability of the patient's plasma to inactivate FVIII of pooled normal plasma. The result is expressed in Bethesda units (BU), one BU being equal to the amount of inhibitor which destroys half (50%) of FVIII in the mixture that was incubated for 2 hours at 37°C. These units of inhibition are plotted and multiplied by the reciprocal of the dilution factor to determine the BU in undiluted plasma [12]. The inhibitor concentration varies from person to person and can also vary within the same person over the course of time. According to the test results of Bethesda, the inhibitors are known as "high titer" (more than 5 BU) or "low degree" (less than 5 BU). Generally, high-titer inhibitors work powerfully to quickly neutralize the clotting factor concentrates, while low titer inhibitors are weaker and act more slowly. However, this is not always the case. Inhibitors are also classified as "low response" or "high response", depending on the strength of the reaction of the immune system of the person to factor concentrates, based on a previous exposure; this is known as anamnestic response. There is a modification of the Bethesda test known as Nijmegen method. This test can determine the strength (title) of the inhibitor. However, the Bethesda / Nijmegen test method is not available in many laboratories because it requires expertise. Unfortunately there is no standardization in the interpretation of these tests and a coefficient of variation exists among different laboratories which can range from 40% to 60% [41]. (Figure 3) [37].

Several factors influence the results of tests for inhibitors, among which are included characteristics of the test(pH, time and temperature), VWF content in the assay system, nature of the control sample and possible presence of interfering factors (lupus anticoagulant and heparin). The study EACH2 [10] showed that had a range of inhibitors titles with values ranging from 4.3 to about 42.4 UB (12.8 Average UB), this being possibly reflecting variability in detection methods. Several immunoassay tests for the detection of inhibitors exists, like ELISA assay. Unfortunately they are not available for clinical use and they only detect IgG antibodies and also are not functional studies; its utility could focus when there is concomitant lupus anticoagulant interference inhibitors. In 2003 Shetty et al., showed that the ELISA assay detected inhibitors in patients with Bethesda Test that have been interpreted as negative, this may be a reflection of the presence of natural antibodies without inhibitory capacity or otherwise, the presence of very low levels of inhibitors that ELISA assay can detect and not Bethesda [42].

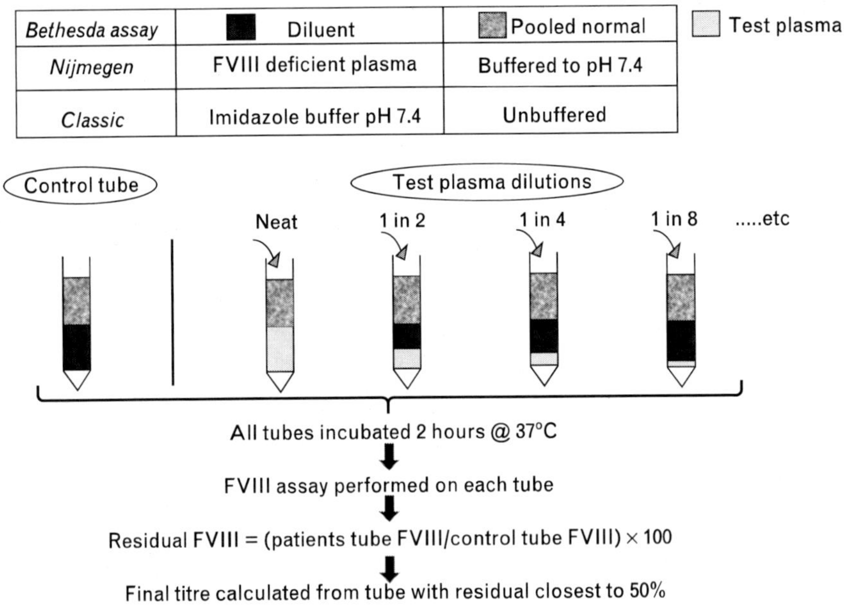

Figure 3. To quantify a factor VIII inhibitor, patient plasma is incubated with a source of FVIII (normal pooled plasma) at 37ºC for 2 hours. A control (FVIII deficient plasma 1 normal pooled plasma) is also incubated at 37ºC for 2 hours. Residual FVIII activity is then measured on both mixtures. The residual FVIII activity of the patient mixture is compared to that of the control mixture (patient/control). If the resulting ratio is <0.40, the patient sample will need to be diluted in either buffer (Bethesda assay) or FVIII deficient plasma (Nijmegen modification). The reciprocal dilution of patient plasma that results in a FVIII activity that is 50% of that of the control mixture is defined as one Bethesda unit (BU). The stronger the inhibitor, the greater the dilution required to allow for expression of the FVIII activity. Reprinted with the permission of the author, from Laboratory identification of factor inhibitors: an update.

5. Treatment Approach

The patient with acquired hemophilia A, with or without bleeding should be managed in a specialized tertiary center. The basics of treatment are based on the following principles; 1) correct the bleeding, 2) eradicate the inhibitor, 3) managing the underlying disease, 4) establishing prophylactic measures to protect against trauma and 5) avoid as far as possible invasive procedures [2].

The risk of bleeding is an individual characteristic of each patient and should always assess the risk on profit starting hemostatic therapy. World literature is clear in recommending that intervention will be require in those patients with: 1) retropharyngeal or retroperitoneal hematomas, 2) muscle bleeding with or without compartment syndrome, 3) intracranial bleeding, 4) lung or digestive tract bleeding, 5) severe hematuria, 6) bleeding in multiple anatomical sites and 7) postoperative bleeding [34]; as already mentioned, it is important to understand that regardless of inhibitor titles or residual activity of FVIII, hemostatic therapy should be initiated as soon as possible. To control bleeding there are multiple therapeutic measures. As first-line treatment is the rFVIIa (Recombinant Factor VIII activated) and aPPC (activated Prothrombin Complex Concentrate) (Table 2). There has always been discussion about what is best agent for bleeding control and therapeutic response. The FENOC study (FEIBA NovoSeven Comparative Study) [43], conducted in patients with alloantibodies was an open, randomized, multicenter prospective analysis where the equivalence of 1 dose of FEIBA (Factor Eight Inhibitor Bypassing Activity) versus 2 doses of rFVIIa was evaluated. During the first two hours seems that FEIBA had greater hemostatic control (53.2% vs. 38.3% p = 0.495), and at 6 hours after administration there was no difference in the hemostatic effect between FEIBA and rFVIIa (80.9% vs. 78.7 % p = 0.059), nor in the resolution of bleeding (76.1% vs. 65.2% p = 0.309). In EACH2 from 15 to 30% of the patients did not require any hemostatic therapy despite the concept that all those with circulating inhibitors are at risk of disease progression and should be treated. 70.5% of patients received haemostatic therapy, 159 of these patients were treated with rFVIIa and 64 patients with APPC, with a percentage of control of bleeding of 92% and 93% respectively; besides, additional hemostatic failure with these agents was lower than those of the second line like the human factor VIII and desmopressin (OR 0.15, 95% CI, 0.04 to 0.53, P = 0.003). The effectiveness of these drugs known as bypassing agents has been demonstrated in other studies [1], indicating that either can be used depending on patient characteristics, costs of local hospital where they are used and the medical familiarity they have with the agent. It is important to note that with the onset of hemostatic therapy there is a thrombotic risk, especially in patients with additional cardiovascular risk factors; EACH2 showed 11 thrombotic events, 7 arterial and 4 venous, despite of this, it is imperative the benefit of early control of bleeding which exceeds the remote risk of thrombosis. Once started hemostatic therapy, especially with rFVIIa, those who do not respond within 24 hours of administration is unlikely to respond after. This has an advantage over the aPPC and is that it can be used concomitantly with tranexamic acid when mucosal bleeding is present without increasing the risk of thrombosis [2]. The human FVIII is less effective than the rFVIIa or FEIBA. No studies have shown that have greater effectiveness. Human FVIII it is characterized by an unpredictable response, and is considered useful if treatment failure to first-line drugs exist and when inhibitor titers are low. It seems that high doses of FVIII associated with immunoadsorption has better hemostatic response. With desmopressin, limitations for it use are similar to those of FVIII, is limited to anecdotal experiences. It could be useful it use in control minor bleeding and when antibody titers are low in association with FVIII levels in 5UI / dL [34].

After starting a therapeutic regimen, follow-up should be based on clinical aspects. Is considered treatment failure when:

1) bleeding persists and there is no change in the loss / unit time blood.
2) hemoglobin levels do not change or even decrease despite its replacement.
3) increase in the size of the bleeding (internal hematoma) based in comparative imaging studies.
4) evidence that the bleeding continues after 48 hours of appropriate therapeutic approach (may be considered 24 hours if the site is critical).
5) presence of new sites of bleeding despite being on optimal treatment.
6) increased of pain associated with hematoma growth despite treatment.

The other mainstay of treatment is to eradicate the inhibitor and thus to avoid the possibility of recurrence. All patients should receive therapy to eradicate the inhibitor even if the initial symptom is mild and even if 25% of patients can have a spontaneous remission [2,10]. In 2003 Delgado et al., [44] developed a meta-analysis that included 249 patients. In that meta-analysis they concluded that the best clinical response was obtained with steroids associated with cyclophosphamide (Prednisolone 1 mg / kg / day plus cyclophosphamide 1 to 2 mg / kg / day for 4 to 6 weeks), with a percentage of complete remission that ranged from 60 to 100% compared with remissions of 30% in those who received only steroids; despite of this there was no difference in overall survival although this could be attributed to the toxic effects of cyclophosphamide. In EACH2 the first line of treatment was only with prednisolone, followed by prednisolone plus cytotoxic agents; indicating that possibly the most important is the individualization of treatment depending on the age of the patients and associated comorbidities.

Rituximab is indicated if there are contraindications to the use of steroids or cyclophosphamide, expert recommendations [2] say that there are good response with Rituximab monotherapy when inhibitor levels are <100UB and when these are > 100UB good response is achieved in conjunction with cytotoxic agents. There are other treatment options such as azathioprine, vincristine, mycophenolate and cyclosporine, which should be considered if after 3-6 weeks there is no increase or decrease in FVIII inhibitor. To date the use of hyperimmune immunoglobulin is not recommended [35]. It is noteworthy in EACH2, that a group of patients used some immune tolerance protocols like Bonn protocol in 9 patients, Budapest protocol in 2 patients and Malmo protocol in 2 patients; although these protocols were first proposed for the treatment of alloantibodies success rates range from 90 to 93% [45,46].

Table 2. Therapeutic approaches for the management of acquired hemophilia

Medication	Initial Dosage	Comments
First line therapy		
rFVIIIa*	90 mcg/kg every 2 hours to control bleeding.	Less frequent doses to avoid recurrence. Those who do not respond to 24 hour of administration unlikely to respond later. It can be used in conjunction with tranexamic acid in bleeding from mucous
aPPC **	50 to 100 mcg / kg BID or TID (Max 200U/kg/day)	Additional doses for persistent bleeding
Second Line therapy		
Human FVIII	Loading dose = Inhibitor titles (UB) x plasma volume (ml) (Usually = Bolo 20-50 IU / Kg) Followed = Bolo 20 to 50 IU / kg TID or QID - 3 to 4mcg / kg / hour	Less effective than rFVIIa or FEIBA Unpredictable response Useful when low inhibitor titers or a 1st line treatment failure. High dose plus immunoadsorption better hemostatic response.
Desmopressin	0.3mcg / kg IV or SC (Max 24mcg)	Similar limitations to the use of human FVIII. Anecdotal experiences. Unpredictable response Tachyphylaxis with repeated doses. Hyponatremia and seizures. It can be useful: small bleeding, low antibody titres and FVIII levels in 5UI / dL
Porcine FVIII	Currently unavailable	
Third line therapy – if first line treatment fails.		
Immunoadsorption and/or plasmapheresis		
Inhibitor eradication		

Table 2. (Continued)

Medication	Initial Dosage	Comments
Prednisone	1mg/kg/day, 4 to 6 weeks	It can be used alone or in combination with cyclophosphamide
Cyclophosphamide	1.5 – 2mg/kg/day, maximum 5 weeks	Possible side effects: 1. Increase the possibility of prostate cancer and renal pathways. 2. Bleeding in the bladder. 3. Dilutional hyponatremia by increasing ADH (antidiuretic hormone or vasopressin) 4. Dysuria, produced by irritation of the drug. 5. Chance of infertility in men and women. 6. Nausea. 7. Neutropenia. 8. Amenorrhea. It should be used in conjunction with prednisolone
Other agents that could be used	Rituximab (375mg/m2 weekly for 4weeks) Azathioprine Cyclosporine Mycophenolate Vincristine Immune tolerance induction (ITI) with FVIII products	

* Recombinant Factor VIII activated (NOVOSEVEN)

** Activated Prothrombin Complex Concentrate (FEIBA contains FVIIa, FIXa and FXa)

Once FVIII levels > 100 IU / dL are met thromboprophylaxis should be started, monitoring should be very close and regular by a multidisciplinary group for the first 12 months. Relapses occur in up to 20% of patients and when this it happens is to be considered search for malignancy if it was not done before. There are some case reports [36] where up to 20% of patients are cured of the inhibitor with solid tumor resection, as has happened in the description of our case. It is likely that this measure will decrease the antigenic load and then humoral control hyperactivity; is possible that those who do not have such favorable response, is because of either advanced or metastatic neoplastic disease. It is recommended in the same way to measure levels of FVIII and look for the presence of inhibitors before an invasive procedure [35].

Conclusion

It is important to be aware that by definition acquired hemophilia is a rare disorder characterized by spontaneous bleeding in a patient with no previous personal or family hemorrhagic history. It is recommended that treating clinicians, when confronted with a case of Acquired Hemophilia perform an though and systematic clinical examination exercise for proper diagnostic and therapeutic approach.

According to the published data, acquired hemophilia is a disorder of biphasic appearance, with better prognosis and response to treatment in young and pregnant patients. In this young group their clinical manifestations are different from congenital hemophilia, as they tends to have more bleeding in skin and abdomen and less in joints. A situation that limits the proper diagnosis is the lack of standardization in laboratory tests; however as clinicians we must bear in mind that in the appropriate setting a prolonged aPTT should make us alert to the possibility of an acquired hemophilia or or the presence of interference inhibitors that is affecting test in vitro as we already mentioned.

Once the diagnosis is confirmed it should be sought for a possible underlying cause for adequate control of the disease and to prevent recurrence. The basis of medical treatment is based on the combined use of immunosuppressive agents and bypassing agents. Immune tolerance protocols appear to be effective but have developed in very small populations and are much more expensive so it is not recommended as first-line therapy.

References

[1] Franchini M, Mannucci PM. Acquired haemophilia A: a 2013 update. *Thromb Haemost.* 2013 Dec;110(6):1114–20.

[2] Collins P, Baudo F, Huth-Kühne A, Ingerslev J, Kessler CM, Castellano MEM, et al., Consensus recommendations for the diagnosis and treatment of acquired hemophilia A. *BMC Res Notes.* 2010;3:161.

[3] Mulliez SMN, Vantilborgh A, Devreese KMJ. Acquired hemophilia: a case report and review of the literature. *Int J Lab Hematol.* 2014 Jun;36(3):398–407.

[4] Tay L, Duncan E, Singhal D, Al-Qunfoidi R, Coghlan D, Jaksic W, et al., Twelve years of experience of acquired hemophilia A: trials and

tribulations in South Australia. *Semin Thromb Hemost.* 2009 Nov;35(8):769–77.

[5] Collins P, Macartney N, Davies R, Lees S, Giddings J, Majer R. A population based, unselected, consecutive cohort of patients with acquired haemophilia A. *Br J Haematol.* 2004 Jan;124(1):86–90.

[6] Collins PW, Hirsch S, Baglin TP, Dolan G, Hanley J, Makris M, et al., Acquired hemophilia A in the United Kingdom: a 2-year national surveillance study by the United Kingdom Haemophilia Centre Doctors' Organisation. *Blood.* 2007 Mar 1;109(5):1870–7.

[7] Green D, Lechner K. A survey of 215 non-hemophilic patients with inhibitors to Factor VIII. *Thromb Haemost.* 1981 Jun 30;45(3):200–3.

[8] Franchini M, Gandini G, Di Paolantonio T, Mariani G. Acquired hemophilia A: a concise review. *Am J Hematol.* 2005 Sep;80(1):55–63.

[9] Franchini M, Lippi G. Acquired factor VIII inhibitors. *Blood.* 2008 Jul 15;112(2):250–5.

[10] Knoebl P, Marco P, Baudo F, Collins P, Huth-Kühne A, Nemes L, et al., Demographic and clinical data in acquired hemophilia A: results from the European Acquired Haemophilia Registry (EACH2). *J Thromb Haemost JTH.* 2012 Apr;10(4):622–31.

[11] Carmona E, Aznar JA, Jorquera JI, Villanueva MJ, Sánchez-Cuenca JM. Detection of two different anti-factor VIII/von Willebrand factor antibodies of the IgA class in a hemophilic patient with a polyclonal factor VIII inhibitor of the IgG class. *Thromb Res.* 1991 Jul 1;63(1):73–84.

[12] Sakurai Y, Takeda T. Acquired Hemophilia A: A Frequently Overlooked Autoimmune Hemorrhagic Disorder. *J Immunol Res.* 2014;2014:320674.

[13] Toschi V, Baudo F. Diagnosis, laboratory aspects and management of acquired hemophilia A. *Intern Emerg Med.* 2010 Aug;5(4):325–33.

[14] Coppola A, Favaloro EJ, Tufano A, Di Minno MND, Cerbone AM, Franchini M. Acquired inhibitors of coagulation factors: part I-acquired hemophilia A. *Semin Thromb Hemost.* 2012 Jul;38(5):433–46.

[15] Hauser I, Lechner K. Solid tumors and factor VIII antibodies. *Thromb Haemost.* 1999 Sep;82(3):1005–7.

[16] Sallah S, Wan JY. Inhibitors against factor VIII in patients with cancer. Analysis of 41 patients. *Cancer.* 2001 Mar 15;91(6):1067–74.

[17] Sallah S, Nguyen NP, Abdallah JM, Hanrahan LR. Acquired hemophilia in patients with hematologic malignancies. *Arch Pathol Lab Med.* 2000 May;124(5):730–4.

[18] Franchini M, Targher G, Manzato F, Lippi G. Acquired factor VIII inhibitors in oncohematology: a systematic review. *Crit Rev Oncol Hematol.* 2008 Jun;66(3):194–9.

[19] Coppola A, Tufano A, Di Capua M, Franchini M. Bleeding and thrombosis in multiple myeloma and related plasma cell disorders. *Semin Thromb Hemost.* 2011 Nov;37(8):929–45.

[20] Meiklejohn DJ, Watson HG. Acquired haemophilia in association with organ-specific autoimmune disease. *Haemoph Off J World Fed Hemoph.* 2001 Sep;7(5):523–5.

[21] Trotta F, Bajocchi G, La Corte R, Moratelli S, Sun LY. Long-lasting remission and successful treatment of acquired factor VIII inhibitors using cyclophosphamide in a patient with systemic lupus erythematosus. *Rheumatol Oxf Engl.* 1999 Oct;38(10):1007–9.

[22] Soriano RM, Matthews JM, Guerado-Parra E. Acquired haemophilia and rheumatoid arthritis. *Br J Rheumatol.* 1987 Oct;26(5):381–3.

[23] Vignes S, Le Moing V, Meekel P, Papo T, Wechsler B, Godeau P. Acquired hemophilia: a rare complication of Sjögren's syndrome. *Clin Exp Rheumatol.* 1996 Oct;14(5):559–60.

[24] Sievert R, Goldstein ML, Surks MI. Graves' disease and autoimmune factor VIII deficiency. *Thyroid Off J Am Thyroid Assoc.* 1996 Jun;6(3):245–7.

[25] Sallah S, Wan JY. Inhibitors against factor VIII associated with the use of interferon-alpha and fludarabine. *Thromb Haemost.* 2001 Oct;86(4):1119–21.

[26] Regina S, Colombat P, Fimbel B, Guerois C, Gruel Y. Acquired inhibitor to factor VIII in a patient with Hodgkin's disease following treatment with interferon-alpha. *Haemoph Off J World Fed Hemoph.* 2001 Sep;7(5):526–7.

[27] Mauser Bunschoten EP, Damen M, Reesink HW, Roosendaal G, Chamuleau RA, van den Berg HM. Formation of antibodies to factor VIII in patients with hemophilia A who are treated with interferon for chronic hepatitis C. *Ann Intern Med.* 1996 Aug 15;125(4):297–9.

[28] Franchini M, Capra F, Nicolini N, Veneri D, Manzato F, Baudo F, et al., Drug-induced anti-factor VIII antibodies: a systematic review. *Med Sci Monit Int Med J Exp Clin Res.* 2007 Apr;13(4):RA55–61.

[29] Dentale N, Fulgaro C, Guerra L, Fasulo G, Mazzetti M, Fabbri C. Acquisition of factor VIII inhibitor after acute hepatitis C virus infection. *Blood. 1*997 Oct 15;90(8):3233–4.

[30] Michiels JJ. Acquired hemophilia A in women postpartum: clinical manifestations, diagnosis, and treatment. *Clin Appl Thromb Off J Int Acad Clin Appl Thromb.* 2000 Apr;6(2):82–6.

[31] Santoro RC, Prejanò S. Postpartum-acquired haemophilia A: a description of three cases and literature review. *Blood Coagul Fibrinolysis Int J Haemost Thromb.* 2009 Sep;20(6):461–5.

[32] Ries M, Wölfel D, Maier-Brandt B. Severe intracranial hemorrhage in a newborn infant with transplacental transfer of an acquired factor VII:C inhibitor. *J Pediatr.* 1995 Oct;127(4):649–50.

[33] Arbuckle MR, McClain MT, Rubertone MV, Scofield RH, Dennis GJ, James JA, et al., Development of autoantibodies before the clinical onset of systemic lupus erythematosus. *N Engl J Med.* 2003 Oct 16;349(16):1526–33.

[34] Collins PW. Therapeutic challenges in acquired factor VIII deficiency. *Hematol Educ Program Am Soc Hematol Am Soc Hematol Educ Program.* 2012;2012:369–74.

[35] Huth-Kühne A, Baudo F, Collins P, Ingerslev J, Kessler CM, Lévesque H, et al., International recommendations on the diagnosis and treatment of patients with acquired hemophilia A. *Haematologica.* 2009 Apr;94(4):566–75.

[36] Sborov DW, Rodgers GM. How I manage patients with acquired haemophilia A. *Br J Haematol.* 2013 Apr;161(2):157–65.

[37] Kershaw G, Favaloro EJ. Laboratory identification of factor inhibitors: an update. *Pathology (Phila).* 2012 Jun;44(4):293–302.

[38] Chang H-H, Chiang B-L. The diagnosis and classification of autoimmune coagulopathy: An updated review. *Autoimmun Rev.* 2014 Apr;13(4–5):587–90.

[39] Kasper CK, Aledort L, Aronson D, Counts R, Edson JR, van Eys J, et al., Proceedings: A more uniform measurement of factor VIII inhibitors. *Thromb Diath Haemorr*h. 1975 Nov 15;34(2):612.

[40] Chang S, Tillema V, Scherr D. A “Percent Correction” Formula for Evaluation of Mixing Studies. *Am J Clin Pathol.* 2002 Jan 1;117(1):62–73.

[41] Favaloro EJ, Verbruggen B, Miller CH. Laboratory testing for factor inhibitors. *Haemoph Off J World Fed Hemoph.* 2014 May;20 Suppl 4:94–8.

[42] Shetty S, Ghosh K, Mohanty D. An ELISA assay for the detection of factor VIII antibodies - comparison with the conventional Bethesda

assay in a large cohort of haemophilia samples. *Acta Haematol.* 2003;109(1):18–22.

[43] Astermark J, Donfield SM, DiMichele DM, Gringeri A, Gilbert SA, Waters J, et al., A randomized comparison of bypassing agents in hemophilia complicated by an inhibitor: the FEIBA NovoSeven Comparative (FENOC) Study. *Blood.* 2007 Jan 15;109(2):546–51.

[44] Delgado J, Jimenez-Yuste V, Hernandez-Navarro F, Villar A. Acquired haemophilia: review and meta-analysis focused on therapy and prognostic factors. *Br J Haematol.* 2003 Apr;121(1):21–35.

[45] Zeitler H, Ulrich-Merzenich G, Hess L, Konsek E, Unkrig C, Walger P, et al., Treatment of acquired hemophilia by the Bonn-Malmo Protocol: documentation of an in vivo immunomodulating concept. *Blood.* 2005 Mar 15;105(6):2287–93.

[46] Nemes L, Pitlik E. New protocol for immune tolerance induction in acquired hemophilia. *Haematologica.* 2000 Oct;85(10 Suppl):64–8.

In: Clotting Disorders
Editor: Jeffrey L. Wilson
ISBN: 978-1-63482-830-7

Chapter 2

Lower Gastrointestinal Bleeding in Children: Etiology and Clinical Management

Francesca Penagini, Chiara Mameli, Giacomo Colella, Dario Dilillo and Gian Vincenzo Zuccotti
Pediatric Department, Ospedale dei Bambini
V. Buzzi, University of Milan, Milan, Italy

Abstract

Gastrointestinal bleeding (GIB) is a relatively common event in the pediatric population, it can potentially occur anywhere in the enteric canal which is highly vascularised. It is important to investigate appropriately every child presenting with GIB, keeping in mind that this phenomenon can be the presenting sign for heterogeneous pathologies with different severity, ranging from benign conditions that require little if any intervention to severe diseases including surgical emergencies, inflammatory bowel disease (IBD) and clotting disorders. The term GIB includes both upper gastrointestinal bleeding (UGIB) and lower gastrointestinal bleeding (LGIB). The former refers to bleeding that originates proximal to the ligament of Treitz, the latter bleeding distal to the ligament of Treitz. The present review chapter focuses on LGIB in children, describing epidemiology, etiology according to children's age and proposes a practical algorithm for clinical management. LGIB represents 0.3% of the referrals to a Pediatric Emergency Department and is usually a benign condition which resolves spontaneously in 80% of cases. However, in approximately 20% of cases it may be the sign of severe disease or potentially life threatening conditions. The etiology of LGIB in pediatric age varies significantly according to the child's age. For example, in neonatal age frequent causes are represented by swallowed maternal blood and surgical emergencies such as necrotizing enterocolitis, malrotation with midgut volvulus and hirschsprung's disease. In infancy (age range 1 month-2 years), the causes are heterogenous ranging from anorectal fissures and allergic proctitis to more severe diseases such as hemolytic uremic syndrome, henoch-schönlein purpura and surgical conditions including intussusception and meckel's diverticulum. In pre-school children (age range 2-5 years) infectious diarrhoea, gastrointestinal polyps and polyposis syndromes are the most common causes of LGIB. In school-aged children and adolescents, the spectrum of disorders with LGIB is similar to that of preschool children, with the exception that IBD often occurs in this age range. Besides the above described diseases which are typical of children in specific age ranges, several clotting disorders may be responsible of LGIB across all pediatric ages.

In fact, coagulopathies (either congenital or acquired) and thrombocytopenias (either idiopathic or secondary), besides presenting more commonly with epistaxis, hematoma's and hemathrosis may more rarely present with acute gastrointestinal bleeding. In the clinical management of LGIB a two-step approach can be proposed. The first step is to assess the general well-being of the patient, and to treat or prevent hemodynamic instability. After assessment of hemodynamic stability and stabilisation of critical patients the second step is to distinguish UGIB from LGIB and if possible to identify the site of GIB. A thorough history, and an accurate physical examination followed by laboratory and imaging tests represent the cornerstone of LGIB work-up.

Introduction

Gastrointestinal bleeding (GIB) is a relatively common event in the pediatric population and may be cause of anxiety for caregivers. GIB can potentially occur anywhere in the enteric canal, which is highly vascularised.

It is important to investigate appropriately every child presenting with GIB, keeping in mind that this phenomenon can be the presenting sign for different pathologies, ranging from benign conditions, that need little if any intervention, to severe diseases, such as surgical emergencies, clotting disorders, and inflammatory bowel disease (IBD).

The term GIB includes both upper gastrointestinal bleeding (UGIB) and lower gastrointestinal bleeding (LGIB). The former refers to bleeding that originates proximal to the ligament of Treitz, while the latter distal to the ligament of Treitz. The present review focuses on LGIB in children.

Epidemiology

LGIB represents 0.3% of the referrals to a Pediatric Emergency Department (ED) [1], it is usually a benign condition which resolves spontaneously in 80% of cases. However, it is always worth investigating to rule out the occurrence of potentially severe diseases. In a pediatric series, on 104 children admitted to the ED for gastrointestinal bleeding 4 (4.2%) had a life threatening condition; 3 where intussusceptions and 1 was a Meckel's diverticulum [1]. Mortality from LGIB is low and usually related to a coexisting pathological state (e.g. vascular malformation, liver disease, portal hypertension). LGIB may present as bloody diarrhea which can be a sign of infectious gastroenteritis. An estimate of the annual incidence of bacterial gastroenteritis presenting with bloody diarrhea in the pediatric population is around 50-75 in 100 000 children [2, 3]. Besides infectious disease, bloody diarrhea is a common presenting symptom of IBD, occurring in about 75% of children with UC and 25% with CD at onset of disease [4].

Definitions

LGIB is a generic term that includes bleeding from the lower gastrointestinal tract of different entity and severity.

Hematochezia is the passage of stools mixed with blood, usually bright red, or blood coated stools. It usually suggests a LGIB, although a massive upper bleeding can also present in this way.

Melena is the passage of pitch black, tarry, foul-smelling stools, it usually indicates a UGIB, although more rarely also a proximal LGIB can have this presentation. More rarely it can be caused by swallowing of blood from a non-gastrointestinal site (e.g., nose, pharynx). Dark stools caused by medications (e.g., iron), foods (e.g., spinach, beetroots) may be mistaken for melena.

Rectal bleeding is blood loss and/or passage of clots, not related to defecation.

Etiology

The etiology of lower gastrointestinal bleeding varies depending upon age.

Neonatal Period

The most common causes of LGIB in the neonatal period are illustrated in Table 1.

Swallowed Maternal Blood

Rectal bleeding in the neonatal period is not a common finding. In first instance it must be confirmed that the blood is fetal in origin and not swallowed maternal blood. This can be done by using the Apt/Downey test. In this test stool is mixed with sodium hydroxide, a change in colour signifies the presence of maternal blood.

Necrotizing Enterocolitis

Necrotizing enterocolitis (NEC) is a severe inflammatory disorder of the intestine. It can involve any segment of the gastrointestinal tract, but most commonly occurs in the distal ileum. The incidence of NEC is about 1 in 1000 live births [5, 6], with over 90% of cases occurring in premature infants and an incidence that tends to increase with decreasing birth weight.

Traditionally, NEC has been described to occur in the second week of life, and almost after start of enteral feeds. Early nonspecific signs include lethargy, apnoea, bradycardia and temperature instability.

Table 1.

Lower gastrointestinal bleeding in newborns
– Swallowed maternal blood
– Necrotizing enterocolitis
– Malrotation with midgut volvulus
– Hirschsprung's disease

These may progress to increased ventilatory requirements and poor perfusion requiring pressure support. Early gastrointestinal tract signs include feeding intolerance, increased gastric residuals, abdominal distension, bilious vomiting and gross or occult blood in stool. As disease progresses, patients may develop abdominal wall tenderness or discoloration and erythema or ecchymosis and palpable distended loops of bowel.

Hirschsprung's Disease

Hirschsprung's disease (HD) is a congenital condition of the distal gastrointestinal tract characterized by the lack of intestinal ganglia. The affected segment acts as a functional obstruction due to the absence of ganglion cells and a failure of smooth muscle to relax. Common initial symptoms are abdominal distention (76-100%), vomiting (69-72%) which can be bilious, as well as delayed passage of meconium [7]. Hirschsprung associated enterocolitis (HAEC) is a serious, life-threatening complication of HD, occurring preoperatively or at the time of diagnosis in 6-26% of cases and post pull-through surgery in 5-42% [8, 9]. There appears to be an increased risk in the first year after surgery and in patients with Down's syndrome [10]. The pathophysiology of HAEC remains poorly understood, the etiology seems to result from various dysfunctions of intestinal homeostasis including mucosal immunity defects, disordered motility, abnormal mucin production, and infection [11]. The major presenting features of HAEC are abdominal distension (83%), explosive diarrhoea (69%), vomiting (51%), fever (34%), lethargy (27%) and rectal bleeding (5%) [12].

Malrotation with Midgut Volvulus

Intestinal malrotation is a congenital anomaly of the rotation of the midgut characterized by an abnormal position of the duodeno-jejunal junction, which may lead life threatening midgut volvulus and bowel necrosis. The majority of patients present in the first year of life with symptoms of acute or chronic obstruction. Infants often (50-75%) develop symptoms within the first month of life presenting with bilious emesis and acute bowel obstruction [13]. Older patients might present with nonspecific gastrointestinal complaints such as recurrent abdominal pain and vomiting, resulting from intermittent volvulus [14].

Signs of bowel ischemia, including abdominal wall erythema, peritonitis, respiratory failure, hematemesis and melena, usually do not manifest until the process is advanced.

Infancy

The most common causes of LGIB in infancy (1 month-2 years) are described in Table 2.

Anorectal Fissures

Anorectal fissure is a longitudinal tear in the distal anal canal. In children it represents a common problem which may occur at any age, but typically presents around 2 years of age. Typical symptoms are rectal bleeding and pain, or crying with defecation. A history of constipation with painful defecation and withholding behaviour is common. The pathogenesis of anal fissures is uncertain, but is postulated to involve internal anal sphincter hypertonia and chronic constipation. It is likely that a mechanical disruption occurs from hard stools leading to secondary constipation from stool avoidance causing a cyclical damage. Diagnosis is done by gentle retraction and external examination of the anal canal. Lesions are often in the posterior midline, but particularly in infants, may be found anywhere in the canal. Most anal fissures will heal spontaneously; when associated with constipation, they respond well to stool softeners and lubricants.

Table 2.

Lower gastrointestinal bleeding in infancy (1 month- 2 years)
– Anorectal fissures
– Allergic colitis
– Intussusception
– Meckel's diverticulum
– Hemolytic Uremic Syndrome (HUS)
– Henoch-Schönlein Purpura (HSP)
– Lymphonodular hyperplasia
– Gastrointestinal duplication

Dietary Protein-Induced Proctitis/Proctocolitis

Dietary protein-induced proctitis/proctocolitis generally manifests during the first months of life, with a mean age at diagnosis of 2 months; cow's milk protein and less frequently, soy protein are the most common triggers [15]. Clinically, it manifests with visible specks or streaks of blood mixed with mucus in stool in an otherwise healthy infant; blood loss is usually minimal, and anemia is rare.

Most infants present while being breastfed, symptoms occur as a result of maternally ingested proteins excreted in breast milk [16, 17]. Nevertheless, the disorder has also been noted in infants who are fed with casein hydrolysed formulas [18]. The differential diagnosis includes causes such as infection and anal fissures. The lack of systemic symptoms and other gastrointestinal symptoms such as vomiting, diarrhoea and failure to thrive help differentiation from other disorders and food allergies.

Evidence for diagnosis is obtained from clinical response to dietary elimination of the causal food protein, hence for breastfed infants maternal restriction of cow's milk is required, and for formula fed infants substitution with a protein hydrolysed formula is suggested. Bleeding is expected to resolve within 72 hours of dietary exclusion of the causal food protein. If maternal manipulations fail to resolve the bleeding a trial of hydrolysed formula may be suggested. If prolonged bleeding persists despite the hydrolysed formula, an aminoacid based formula may be needed. The natural history of the disorder is spontaneous resolution by age 1 or 2 years of age, at that time the causal food protein can be gradually added back to the diet, with close monitoring of visible blood in stools. The recovery rate is approximately

50% at 1 year, 70% at 2 years and 80% at 3 years of age [19]. The mechanism underlying the disorder is not completely understood, but it is seems to be non-IgE mediated, as skin prick tests and fluorescent enzyme immunoassays are characteristically negative in this condition.

Intussusception

Intussusception represents the most common cause of intestinal obstruction in infants, occurring when one portion of small bowel invaginates into a more distal portion of the bowel. Venous congestion and bowel wall edema can cause obstruction of the intestine, and infarction and perforation of the bowel wall can occur.

Around 68-92% of intussusception diagnoses are in children younger than 1 year of age, with a peak incidence in children 3-9 months [20, 21]. Several risk factors have been described such as concurrent respiratory infection (e.g adenovirus), gastroenteritis, Henoch-Schönlein Purpura and lymphonodular hyperplasia. In 2-8% of patients, a recognizable lead point of the intussusception is found, such as Meckel's diverticulum, intestinal polyp, neurofibroma, intestinal duplication, hemangioma, or malignant condition such as lymphoma. Intussusceptions are most often ileocolic, less commonly cecocolic, and rarely exclusively ileal. In typical cases there is sudden onset, in a previously well child, of severe paroxysmal colicky pain that recurs at frequent intervals and is accompanied by straining efforts with legs and knees flexed and loud cries. The infant may initially be comfortable and play normally between the paroxysms of pain; but if the intussusception is not reduced, the infant becomes progressively weaker and lethargic. Vomiting occurs in most cases and is usually more frequent in the early phase; in the later stage it may become bile stained. Around 60% of infants pass a stool containing red blood and mucus, the classic red-currant-jelly stool. Palpation of the abdomen usually reveals a slightly tender sausage-shaped mass, which may increase in size and firmness during a paroxysm of pain. Abdominal ultrasound is typically performed when intussusception is suspected. Air, hydrostatic (saline) and, less often, water-soluble contrast enemas have replaced barium examinations and are useful for both diagnosis and reduction of intussusception [22].

Meckel's Diverticulum

Meckel's diverticulum (MD) is the most prevalent congenital abnormality of the gastrointestinal tract. This anomaly is due to the incomplete obliteration of the omphalomesenteric duct during the 7th week of gestation and is classically located 50-75 cm from the ileocecal valve. MD remains mostly asymptomatic in affected individuals, there is 4-6% probability of symptomatic presentations [23]. Gastrointestinal bleeding is the major clinical finding in children with symptomatic MD. The incidence rate for this complication has been recorded as high as 50% [24]. The primary reason for the gastrointestinal bleeding has been associated with ectopic tissue, gastric tissue in 60-65% of cases [25]. Less often, a MD is associated with partial or complete bowel obstruction. The most common mechanism of obstruction occurs when the diverticulum acts as the lead point of an intussusception.

The most sensitive study for diagnosis of MD is the Meckel radionuclide scan, which is performed after intravenous infusion of technetium-99m pertechnetate, permitting visualization of the diverticulum.

Hemolytic Uremic Syndrome

Hemolytic uremic syndrome (HUS) is characterized by the acute onset of the triad: microangiopathic hemolytic anemia, renal injury and thrombocytopenia. An acute enteritis with diarrhea caused by Shiga-like toxin-producing Escherichia coli 0157:H7 precedes 80% or more of HUS cases in developed countries [26]. HUS is most common in children younger than 4 years of age. The onset is usually preceded by a gastroenteritis characterized by fever, vomiting, abdominal pain and diarrhea that is initially watery but then becomes bloody. Sudden onset of pallor, irritability, weakness, lethargy, and oliguria usually occurs 5-10 days after the initial gastrointestinal illness.

Henoch-Schönlein Purpura

Henoch-Schönlein purpura (HSP) is a vasculitis of small vessels with cutaneous and systemic complications. HSP represents the most common systemic vasculitis in childhood, occurring typically in children aged 2 -8 years. HSP is mediated by immune deposits (typically IgA), resulting in necrosis of the wall of small and medium-sized arteries with extravasation of erythrocytes and infiltration of tissue with neutrophils, a picture called leukocytoclastic vasculitis. Palpable purpura is the presenting sign in 57-69% of patients, with lesions occurring in crops and fading within 7-10 days [27]. Joint involvement occurs in 43-82% of cases with symmetrical oligoarthritis (ankles, feet, knees) and renal involvement occurs in 32-54% of cases, mainly with hematuria [28]. Gastrointestinal involvement occurs in 51-74% of patients with HSP, presenting with abdominal pain, nausea, vomiting of bleeding [29]. The abdominal pain is characteristically colicky and localized to the periumbilical and epigastric regions, it worsens after meals similar to bowel angina or ischemia. There is occult or, less commonly, overt bleeding in 18-52% of patients with HSP [30]. The small intestine is the most frequently involved site in the gastrointestinal tract due to its predilection toward ischemic injury.

Intussusception (most frequently ileo-ileal) is the most common surgical complication of HSP in childhood, occurring in 0.7-13.6% of patients [31].

Lymphonodular Hyperplasia

Lymphonodular hyperplasia (LNH) of the colon and/or terminal ileum is a frequent endoscopic finding in children evaluated for lower gastrointestinal bleeding [32]. Biopsy specimens from children with LNH contain increased number of lymphoid follicles and larger follicles, mucosal inflammation and epithelial thinning and ulceration overlying enlarged follicles.

Because LNH disrupts the normal mucosa, it leads to mucosal thinning and predisposes to ulceration, which may cause hematochezia. Blood loss is usually minimal and painless but is present in multiple stools.

An association between LNH and gastrointestinal food allergy has been described [33]. In a study conducted by Iacono et al. [34], LNH was identified in 73 (30%) of 245 children who underwent ileocolonoscopy for gastrointestinal symptoms.

LNH was the only finding in 52 of 73 cases (71%). In 43 of these 52 patients a diagnosis of cow's milk or multiple food hypersensitivity was made. The patients with LNH and food hypersensitivity presented with hematochezia more frequently than those without LNH ($p<0.0001$).

Gastrointestinal Duplication

Enteric duplication (ED) is a rare congenital anomaly that can occur anywhere along the length of the gastrointestinal tract, with the ileum representing the most common site of occurrence [35].

The pathogenesis is still vaguely understood, however, errors in canalization or embryologic connection between the developing gut and neural tube have been postulated. The clinical presentations may be vague, diverse, and varied depending on their size, localization and mucosal lining [36].

These include nausea, vomiting, abdominal distention, dysphagia and dyspepsia. ED can cause bowel obstruction by compressing the adjacent intestinal lumen, or they can act as the lead point of an intussusception or a site for a volvulus. If they are lined by acid- secreting mucosa, they can cause ulceration, perforation and hemorrhage.

Table 3.

Lower gastrointestinal bleeding in pre-school children (2-5 years)
– Infectious diarrhea – Polyps

Preschool Children

The most common causes of LGIB in preschool children (2-5 years) are described in Table 3.

Infectious Diarrhea

A number of pathogens can cause lower gastrointestinal bleeding in children. Infection should be considered in children presenting with bleeding accompanied by other symptoms such as fever, abdominal pain and tenesmus. The most common infectious agents causing bloody diarrhea, as well as clinical presentation and recommended therapy are described in table 4 [37, 38, 39].

Polyps and Polyposis Syndromes

Gastrointestinal polyps are common during childhood and most often present with painless rectal bleeding. The most frequent condition is an isolated colonic lesion, which isn't a sign of any underlying genetic disorder, nor do they carry the risk of gastrointestinal cancer. However, occasionally polyps may occur in the context of a genetic polyposis disorder characterized by an increase in life-time risk of cancer in the gastrointestinal tract and other organ systems [40].

- *Juvenile polyps (JP)* are commonly encountered in pediatric practice and typically present in children aged between 2 and 5 years with intermittent, painless rectal bleeding. There is a predominance in the male gender. JP can be found throughout the colon, but predominate in the rectosigmoid region; occasionally they might present as prolapsing rectal lesions and rarely with abdominal pain caused by intussusception. Macroscopically they typically are pedunculated, lobular lesions, often with ulcerated surface and covered in granulation tissue that easily bleeds. Most JP are hamartomatous, non-neoplastic and only rarely show dysplastic changes. Histology is characterized by normal glandular tissue with dilated, mucin-filled cystic glands and a dense infiltrate of inflammatory cells. JP with an adenomatous histology strongly suggest an underlying genetic polyposis syndrome. The preferred method for diagnosis and treatment is pancolonoscopy with polypectomy.
- *Juvenile polyposis syndrome (JPS)* is a rare autosomal dominant condition characterized by the occurrence of multiple JP in the gastrointestinal tract. The entire gastrointestinal tract is usually affected, and the prognosis is related to the severity and extent of gastrointestinal involvement. Compared with patients with solitary juvenile polyps, patients with JPS not only have more polyps but are also more likely to have right-side polyps, polyps with adenomatous change, and anemia [41]. Patients with features suggestive of JPS should have surveillance colonoscopy with random biopsies of polyps and flat mucosa every 2 years [42].
- *Peutz-Jeghers Syndrome (PJS).* Peutz-Jeghers Syndrome is a rare genetic disorder with four major features: 1) multiple gastrointestinal hamartomatous polyps, 2) melanin pigmentation of the skin and mucus membranes, 3) autosomal-dominant mode of inheritance, and

4) significant risk for malignancy in multiple organs. Multiple, peduncolated polyps are found throughout the gastrointestinal tract but most frequently arise in the small bowel (60-90%) and colon (50-64%) [43].

- *Familial adenomatous polyposis (FAP).* In children, gastrointestinal adenomas are almost always associated with hereditary adenomatous polyposis syndromes. FAP is the most common of the adenomatous polyposis syndromes. It is an autosomal dominant condition in which there is a defect in the APC gene on chromosome 5q21. Patients with FAP typically have multiple adenomas throughout the large bowel- usually more than 100 and sometimes more than a 1000. Polyps begin to appear in childhood or adolescence and increase in number with age [44].

Table 4.

Agent	Transmission	Clinical presentation	Therapy
Non-typhoid Salmonella	Ingestion of contaminated raw-meat, poultry, eggs.	Nausea, vomiting, crampy abdominal pain, watery and/or bloody diarrhea.	-Ceftriaxone 75mg/kg/day OD* for 7 days. IV or IM -Ampicillin100mg/kg/day every 6 hrs for 7 days PO**
Shigella	Ingestion of contaminated food (often salads) and water.	Severe abdominal pain, high fever, vomiting, painful defecation. Diarrhea initially watery and subsequently bloody.	-Ampicillin100mg/kg/day every 6 hrs for 7 days PO. -Azithromycin 10mg/kg/day OD for 3 days PO. -Ceftriaxone 75mg/kg/day OD for 7 days. IV or IM.
Campylobacter	Ingestion of contaminated water or food (poultry, raw milk) or transmission from pets (cats, dogs, hamsters) and farm animals.	Fever, vomiting, malaise, myalgia, abdominal pain. Watery and subsequently bloody diarrhoea.	Erythromycin 50 mg/kg/day in 4 divided doses for 5-7 days PO. -Azithromycin 10mg/kg/day OD for 3 days PO.
Clostridium difficile	Altered bowel flora, antimicrobial therapy (ampicillin, 2nd and 3rd generation cephalosporins, clindamycin)	Vary widely: asymptomatic colonization, mild self-limited diarrhea, watery diarrhea with occult blood, pseudomembranous colitis (bloody diarrhea, fever, abdominal pain, nausea, vomiting)	-Metronidazole 20-40mg/kg/day every 6-8 hrs for 7-10days PO -Vancomycin 25-40mg/kg/day every 6hrs for 7-10 days PO.
Yersinia	Ingestion of contaminated food or water, animal contact (domestic and farm animals) and contaminated blood products.	Acute enterocolitis: fever, watery and/or bloody diarrhea, abdominal pain. In older children mesenteric lymphadenitis that may mimic appendicitis.	Ampicillin100mg/kg/day every 6 hrs for 7 days PO. -Azithromycin 10mg/kg/day OD for 3 days PO. -Ceftriaxone 75mg/kg/day OD for 7 days. IV or IM

*OD: once daily, **PO: per os.

School Aged Children and Adolescents

The spectrum of disorders in school-aged children and adolescents with LGIB is similar to that of preschool children, with the exception that Inflammatory Bowel Disease (IBD) often presents in this age range.

Inflammatory Bowel Disease

The term inflammatory bowel disease (IBD) includes two distinctive clinical entities characterized by chronic intestinal inflammation: Crohn's disease (CD) and ulcerative colitis (UC). Whilst the former may involve any region of the alimentary tract from the mouth to the anus, the latter is limited to the colon and usually begin distally in the rectum and extends proximally for a variable distance. The clinical course of these disorders are typically marked by remission and relapse, often without apparent explanation. It is estimated that 25-30% of IBD develops during childhood and adolescence [45]. Bloody diarrhea, urgency, cramping abdominal pain, tenesmus and nocturnal bowel movements are common in UC. The clinical symptoms of CD may vary according to disease behaviour: either inflammatory or structuring/fibrostenosing. Disease phenotype often changes as duration of disease lengthens; inflammatory tends to evolve to structuring. Patients with small bowel disease are more likely to have an obstructive pattern (most commonly right lower quadrant pain), while those with colonic disease are more likely to have symptoms resulting from inflammation (bloody diarrhea, cramping abdominal pain). Systemic signs and symptoms are more common in CD than in UC. Fever, malaise, and easy fatigability are common. Unique to pediatric-onset disease is the potential for linear growth impairment as a complication of undertreated inflammation [46].

Rare Causes of LGIB in Children

Angiodysplasia

Angiodysplasia, a vascular ectasia, is recognized as an important cause of lower gastrointestinal bleeding in the elderly; however, in pediatric population there is little experience [47]. They can occur in any segment of the gastrointestinal tract, the right hemicolon and cecum are the most common sites in adults [48]. A retrospective study conducted by Chuang et al. [49] evaluated clinical manifestations, images, and treatments of angiodysplasia, diagnosed by computed tomographic angiography (CTA) in 18 children aged 0-18 years. The mean age at time of diagnosis was 7.1 years and the patients were predominantly males. The most common symptom was anemia (94.4%), followed by abdominal pain (55.6%), hematochezia (50.0%), melena (50.0%), and infection (50.0%).

The most common affected areas were the ascending colon and terminal ileum (61.1%). Six patients (33.3%) underwent operation to reset the affected segments because of recurrent bleeding and unstable hemodynamic status. Four of them were compatible with angiodysplasia by confirmation of histology. Endoscopy and angiography are the standard diagnostic modalities for angiodysplasia; however, they are invasive tests. CTA is a sensitive, specific, and minimally invasive tool for the diagnosis of angiodysplasia [50, 51].

Solitary Rectal Ulcer Syndrome

Solitary rectal ulcer syndrome (SRUS) is a benign and chronic disorder well known in young adults. In children, SRUS is relatively uncommon but troublesome and easily misdiagnosed with other common disease [52, 53, 54]. It is often related to prolonged excessive straining or abnormal defecation and clinically presents as rectal bleeding, copious mucus discharge, feeling of incomplete defecation, and rarely rectal prolapse. Rectal hypersensitivity leading to the persistent desire to defecate and sensation of incomplete evacuation may have a role in pathophysiology of SRUS [55]. Suresh et al. [56] have evaluated 325 children aged < 18 years during 8 years for various indications such as bleeding, polyp and anal fissure. Twenty-two (6.8%) children were diagnosed with SURS and ranged in age from 18 months to 18 years (median age 10 years). The best approach to treatment starts with family reassurance, regulation of toilet habits, avoidance of straining and encouragement of a high-fibre diet [55].

Clotting Disorders

Lower gastrointestinal bleeding can also be a sign of clotting disorder, including platelet and coagulation defects. Even though these disorders typically present with mucocutaneous and joint bleeds such as petechie, purpura, ecchymosis, epistaxis and hemarthrosis respectively, in severe cases they may manifest with life-threatening mucosal hemorrhages of the gastrointestinal and cerebrovascular systems. Clotting disorders are numerous and in terms of etiology can be hereditary or acquired. In children, the most common bleeding disorders are hereditary such as Wiskott-Aldrich syndrome (WAS).

Among the acquired clotting disorders, the most common is Immune thrombocytopenia (ITP) which typically occurs in otherwise well children following an acute viral infection.

Platelet Disorders That May Present with LGIB

Platelet disorders can present with gastrointestinal bleeding when the platelet defect is severe. These disorders include both quantitative and qualitative platelet defects. The most common platelet disorders in children are illustrated in table 5.

Table 5.

Platelet disorders	
Thrombocytopenia	*Decreased platelet survival* Idiopathic thrombocytopenic purpura Hemolytic uremic syndrome Wiskott-Aldrich syndrome Disseminated intravascular coagulation *Decreased platelet production* Malignancies (leukemia, neuroblastoma) Sepsis Aplastic anemia *Platelet sequestration* Congestive splenomegaly
Disorders of platelet function	*Congenital* Glanzmann's thrombasthenia Bernard-Soulier syndrome *Acquired* Drug induced: aspirin

Idiopathic Thrombocytopenic Purpura

Idiopathic thrombocytopenic purpura (ITP) is an immune-mediated condition characterized by transiently low platelets usually following an acute viral infection in children. One of the striking features of pediatric ITP is the low rate of bleeding, even if platelet count is persistently $< 10 \times 10^9$/l.

From a prospective registry performed by the Intercontinental Childhood ITP Study Group (ICIS) the percentage of children with ITP presenting with severe hemorrhage (epistaxis, melena, menorrhagia and intracranial hemorrhage) at diagnosis is very low, approximately 2.9 %. Overall, in children ITP gastrointestinal bleeding is rare.

Wiskott-Aldrich Syndrome

Wiskott-Aldrich syndrome (WAS) is an X-linked primary immunodeficiency disorder characterized by the "classic triad" of eczema, thrombocytopenia, and severe and often recurrent infections. The gene responsible for WAS is located on the short arm of the X chromosome and encodes for the WAS protein (WASp) which is involved in several intracellular signalling events in nonerythroid hematopoietic cells, including the process of platelet formation, activation, and associated cytoskeletal remodeling. Perturbation in the function and/or the expression of WASp is correlated with the spectrum of clinical findings of "classic" WAS, including defects in platelet production (abnormal platelet formation) and function with diminished platelet survival [57]. Thrombocytopenia in patients with WAS is almost a constant feature, while the severity is variable. Around 50% of patients with WAS present with severe thrombocytopenia with platelet count < 20,000/μL [58]. The degree of platelet depletion determines the severity of bleeding complications that occur in more than 80% of WAS patients: petechie, ecchymoses, easy bruising and epistaxis are frequent manifestations in the mild forms; in more severe cases life-threatening gastrointestinal bleeding and intracranial hemorrhage may occur. Even though the current accepted curative approach for patients with WAS is represented by hematopoietic stem cell transplantation (HSCT), other approaches can be used in addition such as platelet transfusions or thrombopoietin mimetic drugs for patients with clinically severe bleeding.

Glanzmann's Thrombasthenia

Glanzmann thrombastenia (GT) is a rare autosomal recessive bleeding syndrome affecting the megakaryocyte lineage and characterized by lack of platelet aggregation. The molecular basis is linked to quantitative and/or qualitative abnormalities of αIIbβ3 integrin, the receptor that mediates the incorporation of platelets into an aggregate or thrombus at the site of blood vessel injury. GT has a wide clinical spectrum: some patients have only minimal bruising while others have frequent, severe and potentially fatal hemorrhages.

Purpura, epistaxis, gingival hemorrhage, and menorrhagia are common presenting features, but also gastrointestinal bleeding and hematuria may occur and be severe and potentially fatal [59].

Coagulation Disorders That May Present with LGIB

In pediatric age, the most common coagulation disorders are the congenital forms represented by von Willebrand syndrome and hemophilia A and B (table 7).

Von Willebrand Disease

Von Willebrand disease (vWD) arises from deficiency and/or defects of von Willebrand factor (VWF), a multimeric adhesive plasma protein essential for effective primary hemostasis. Gastrointestinal bleeding in vWD is uncommon and the causes are usually the same as in patients without a bleeding disorder, except for angiodysplastic and occult bleeding which are more frequent in vWD patients compared to the general population. In an international survey undertaken to investigate the frequency of the association between vWD and angiodysplasia, a total of 4503 patients with vWD from 297 centres were studied. The incidences of angiodysplasia were 0% for type 1, 2% for type 2, 4.5% for type 3 and 11.7% for the acquired for of vWD. An important finding was that angiodysplastic bleeding only affected patients with type 2 and type 3 vWD [60].

Inherited Hemophilia

Hemophilia A (deficiency in factor VIII) and hemophilia B (deficiency in factor IX) are the most common serious congenital coagulation factor deficiencies which are inherited as a sex-linked recessive pattern.

Table 7.

Coagulation disorders	
Congenital	Hemophilia A (Factor VIII), Hemophilia B (Factor IX) Von Willebrand disease
Acquired	Disseminated intravascular coagulation Vitamin K deficiency Liver disease Warfarin therapy Renal disease

The genetic mutations cause a quantitative decrease in protein expression, a qualitative decrease in protein activity or both. Disease classification is based on the residual factor level, which correlates to bleeding symptoms. The disease is defined as mild when the factor activity is above 5%, in this case bleeding generally occurs following a significant trauma or surgery. In moderate disease, the residual factor activity is around 1-5% and bleeding tends to occur following a mild trauma or surgery. In severe disease, the residual factor activity is < 1% and bleeding generally occurs spontaneously or after a mild trauma. Hemophilia A is more common, occurring in 1:5000 male births, whereas hemophilia B occurs in 1:30,000 male births. Although the typical presenting signs of hemophilia are excessive bruising, intramuscular hematomas and hemarthrosis occurring during the first year of life when a child starts crawling or walking, potentially any type of bleeding is possible in hemophilia, including mucosal bleeding in gastrointestinal system [61].

Diagnosis

In the clinical management of LGIB a three-step approach can be proposed: 1) evaluation of hemodynamic stability and stabilization of patient; 2) Identification of a local cause of bleeding vs. a clotting disorder; 3) Differentiation of UGIB from LGIB.

The first step is represented by stabilization of the patient by assessing the general well-being of the child, treating or preventing hemodynamic instability. An increased heart rate is the first clinical sign to indicate depletion of the blood volume, hypotension and delayed capillary refill time (>3 seconds in children and >1 second in newborn) are also reliable but may not appear immediately. Change in blood pressure with position (decrease of 20 mmHg from supine to sit or standing position) indicates severe blood loss (estimated in 30%) [62]. After assessment of hemodynamic stability, monitor vital parameters: respiratory rate, oxygen saturation, body temperature. In case of signs and symptoms of severe blood loss, administer 10 ml/kg of 0.9% saline within 20 minutes. When estimating blood loss it is important to keep in mind that the quantity of blood reported in stools may lead to underestimation, since a large quantity may still be inside the lumen.

After first assessment and stabilization of critical patients the second step is to identify whether bleeding is due to a local cause or result of a systemic bleeding disorder. The third and last step is to distinguish UGIB from a LGIB and identify the specific site of bleeding.

In performing steps two and three, a thorough history and physical examination are in most cases sufficient for clinical diagnosis. When the clinical presentation is still not clear, laboratory and instrumental tests may be of aid in the work-up process.

History

A thorough history is useful to gather information on the type and entity of blood loss. Family history for inflammatory bowel disease, polyposis or inherited bleeding disorders should be investigated. An accurate description of the event is extremely important because it can raise suspicion of the potential site of bleeding. Table 8 illustrates the most important aspects to focus on, when collecting history of LGIB.

Table 8.

Family history – Family history for: IBD, familial polyposis syndromes, bleeding disorders.
Onset and pattern of LGIB – Acute bleeding refers to a clinically relevant episode with fast onset as well as fast remission, that usually occurs spontaneously. In more severe cases it may be associated to hemodynamic instability – Acute-recurrent bleeding refers to the recurrence of multiple episodes like the one cited above – Occult chronic bleeding refers to a non clinically apparent blood loss, discovered through occult blood test. – Obscure bleeding refers to a recurrent, persistent blood loss whose origin can't be explained after appropriate diagnostic management

Characteristics of LGIB – Colour of the blood: bright red blood usually indicates a more distal bleeding, while black, maroon blood stains or clots are usually come usually from a more proximal location. – Consistency and aspect of the stools: hard stools streaked with little fresh blood may indicate stipsis. On the other hand, bloody diarrhoea can show during bacterial intestinal infections or IBD – Blood only on toilet paper after bowel movements: it is a common presentation of bleeding from anal fissure. – Blood dripping from the anus, not related to defecation: anorectal bleed is more suggestive of IBD or a surgical anomaly (e.g. Meckel's diverticulum)
Associated signs and symptoms – Fever, abdominal pain, diarrhoea, vomiting, weight loss, fatigue: suspect a systemic disease. – Bleeding from other sites (skin, mucous membranes, soft tissues, muscles, joints, urinary tract): petechie, purpura, ecchymosis, easy bruising, hemarthrosis, soft tissue hematomas, hematuria and intracranial hemorrhage.
Others – Recent travels to developing countries: higher risk for gastrointestinal infectious diseases from polluted water or food. – Rule out conditions that mimic a GIB such as bleeding from non-gastrointestinal sites (posterior epistaxis, nose and throat surgical operations, dental procedures), swallowing blood from a maternal wound or fissure in the breastfed infant, drugs and foods that may colour the stools (iron, dyes, beetroot, spinach).

Physical Examination

An accurate physical examination can identify signs suggestive for specific etiologics (Table 8).

Laboratory Studies

Blood Tests

Full hemogram (hemoglobin, hematocrit, total and differential leukocyte counts): checking anemia is the first priority in any bleeding. Hematocrit is an unreliable index of the severity of acute bleeding since compensatory hemodilution can take up to hours to manifest.

Low Mean Corspuscular Volume (MCV) of red blood cells may suggest a chronic and slow blood loss. Platelet count and coagulation profile are useful to rule out the hemostasis defects. Even if rarely, thrombocytopenia may result from EDTA induced clumping of platelets: examination of a peripheral smear will confirm the presence of platelet clumps.

A low hemoglobin may be secondary to the underlying bleed. However, anemia disproportionate to bleeding may suggest red cell destruction, bone marrow failure or leukemia. White blood cell count provides information suggestive of an infectious cause, sepsis or leukemia.

Table 8.

Skin inspection – Oro-buccal pigmentation: sign suggestive of Peutz-Jeger's syndrome – Petechie, bruising: defects of hemostasis, vasculitis (Henoch-Schönlein purpura) – Hemangiomas: congenital vascular anomalies can be the source of bleeding in the gastrointestinal tract – Atopic dermatitis: may be related to milk allergy – Erythema nodosum, pyoderma gangrenosus, clubbing: skin manifestations of chronic inflammation, such as in IBD – Spiders, splinters: sings of portal hypertension
Abdominal examination – Sausage shape mass: especially in correspondence of the transverse colon, may be palpable in some cases of intussusception – Abdominal tenderness: gastroenteritis, IBD, intussusception, volvolus and other surgical emergencies
Perineal inspection – Anal fissures: the most common cause of mild bleeding. Mostly due to constipation, but always consider trauma and sexual abuse – Skin tags, fistule: signs of chronic inflammation; they often occur in IBD
Rectal exploration – This procedure should always be performed during the evaluation of LGIB. It can show hemorrhoids, as well as foreign body, another possible etiology not to forget.

Alteration of renal function (creatinine) may be a sing of kidney injury and lead to diagnosis of hemolytic uremic syndrome (HUS). C-reactive protein (CRP) and Erythrocyte sedimentation rate (ESR) are markers of systemic inflammation; they are usually found increased in IBD and infectious gastroenteritis.

Specific IgE dosage / skin prick test: if an allergy to food is suspected, these test has high, comparable sensitivity to diagnose allergies. It is important always to correlate to the clinical presentation because studies showed how many children who are positive to specific IgE were then negative to a challenge test.

A peripheral smear provides valuable information about platelet size, morphology and presence of clumping. Giant sized platelets are commonly observed in ITP or inherited disorders such as Bernard Soulier syndrome. Wiskott-Aldrich syndrome is characterized by microthrombocytopenia.

Schistocytes may suggest microangiopathic hemolytic anemia, observed in hemolytic uremic syndrome, thrombotic thrombocytopenic purpura or sepsis.

Coagulation assay is important to identify defects of either the intrinsic and extrinsic pathways of coagulation. Prothrombin time (PT) is prolonged due to deficiency of extrinsic pathway (tissue factor, factor VII) or common pathway factors (II, V, X, and fibrinogen). PTT is prolonged due to deficiency of intrinsic pathway (VIII, IX, XI or XII), common pathway factors, or in presence of inhibitors e.g. lupus anticoagulant and heparin). In a child with suspected coagulation disorder, result of an abnormal PT or PTT should be followed by a mixing study.

This aids in differentiating between a clotting factor deficiency and the presence of an inhibitor (e.g. lupus anticoagulant or antibodies to factor). Patient's plasma is mixed in a 1:1 ratio with normal pooled plasma, and the abnormal test is repeated. Normalization of clotting test (PT or PTT) following a 1:1 dilution with normal pooled plasma indicates deficiency of a factor. Majority of inhibitors will not be effectively diluted following the addition of normal pooled plasma, hence an abnormal test after dilution indicates the presence of an inhibitor. When a coagulation factor deficiency is suggested by clinical history, a specific coagulation-factor assay should be performed to confirm the diagnosis.

Stool Tests

Stool examinations are indicated in children with fever and signs of infectious colitis, in this setting culture for bacteria and search for parasites and ova cysts are recommended.

Fecal calprotectin: a recent marker of intestinal inflammation. It has high sensitivity although lack of specificity. It is therefore useful to rule out diseases that cause gastrointestinal inflammation, in first instance IBD.

Imaging and Endoscopy

Small bowel ultrasound: a highly sensitive method for the diagnosis of intestinal inflammation, indicated by free abdominal fluid, enlarged lymph nodes and increased thickness of the intestinal mucosa. It can also be used to rule out intussusceptions, although it requires a well trained, experienced operator.

Plain radiograph: although it has a limited role in the emergency evalutation of LGIB, it can be useful in patients with abdominal distension to diagnose intestinal obstruction/perforation. It can also be helpful for the search of foreign bodies.

Nuclear scan with technetium 99m: also known as Meckel Scan, for its high sensitivity and specificity (78.6-97% and 70.4-100% respectively) [63] for the localization of the ectopic mucosa in the Meckel's diverticulum.

A nuclear scan with marked red blood cells can be used in the detection of small bleeding (up to 0,1 ml/min) [64]. Colonoscopy: this technique has an important diagnostic role as well as a therapeutic one. It is possible to burn bleeding vessels, take biopsies and remove polyps.

Usually the procedure in children needs total sedation and an experienced crew, specialized in the pediatric patient.

Figure 1 shows the proposed algorithm for differential diagnosis of gastrointestinal bleeding in infants and children.

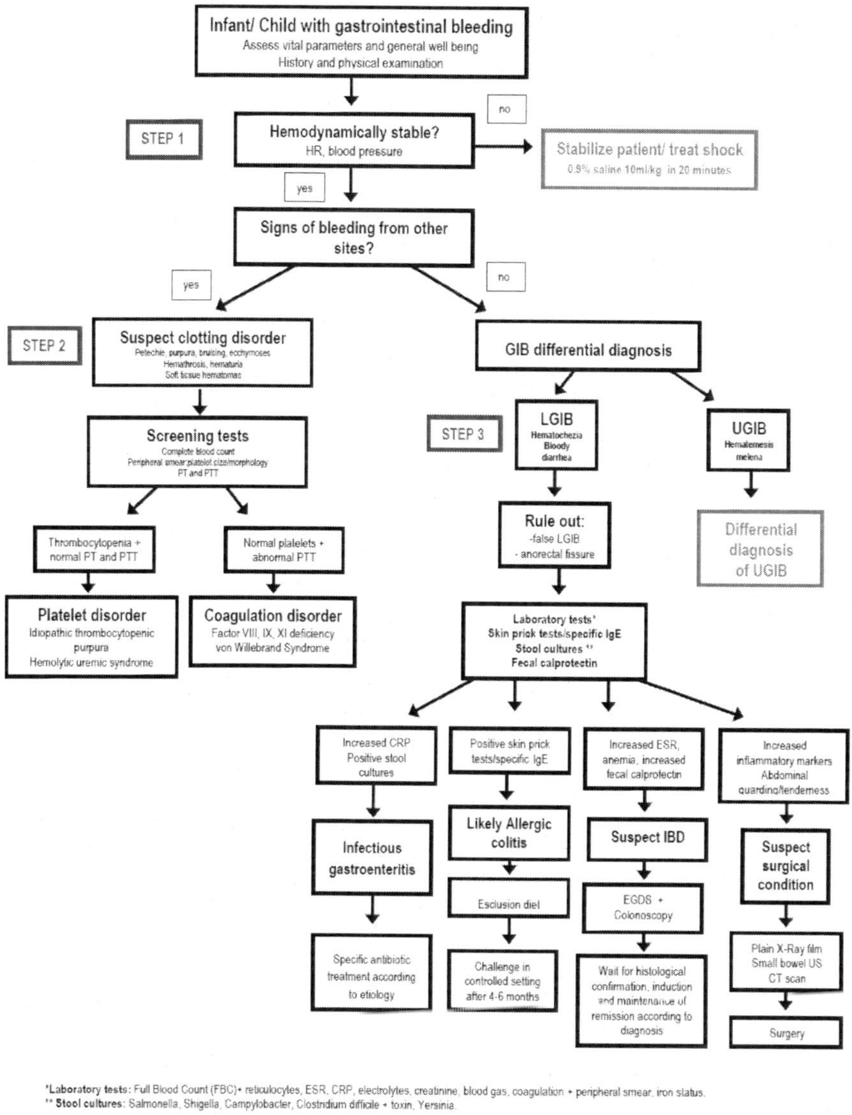

*Laboratory tests: Full Blood Count (FBC) + reticulocytes, ESR, CRP, electrolytes, creatinine, blood gas, coagulation + peripheral smear, iron status.

**Stool cultures: Salmonella, Shigella, Campylobacter, Clostridium difficile + toxin, Yersinia.

Figure 1. Differential diagnosis of gastrointestinal bleeding in infants and children.

References

[1] Teach, S. J., Fleisher, G. R. Rectal bleeding in the pediatric emergency department. *Ann. Emerg. Med.* 1994; 23: 1252.

[2] Wheeler, J. G., Sethi, D., Cowden, J. M., Wall, P. G., Rodrigues, L. C., Tompkins, D. S., et al. Study of infectious intestinal disease in England: rates in the community, presenting to general practice, and reported to national surveillance. The Infectious Intestinal Disease Study Executive. *BMJ* 1999; 318: 1046-50.

[3] Murphy, M. S. Management of bloody diarrhoea in children in primary care. *BMJ* 2008; 336: 1010-5.

[4] Sawczenko, A., Sandhu, B. K. Presenting features of inflammatory bowel disease in Great Britain and Ireland. *Arch. Dis. Child* 2003; 88: 995-1000.

[5] Llanos, A. R., et al. Epidemiology of neonatal necrotising enterocolitis: A population-based study. *Pediatr. Epidemiol.* 2002; 16: 342-349.

[6] Holman, R. C., et al. Necrotising enterocolitis hospitalizations among neonates in the United States. *Pediatr. Perinat. Epidemiol.* 2006; 20: 498-506.

[7] Koh, C. R., Yong, T. L., Fenton, E. J. Hirschprung disease: A regional experience. *ANZ J. Surg.* 2008; 78: 1023-1027.

[8] Vieten, D., Spicer, R. Enterocolitis complicating Hirschprung's disease. *Semin. Pediatr. Surg.* 2004; 13: 263-272.

[9] Ruttenstock, E., Puri, P. Systematic review and meta-analysis of enterocolitis after one-stage transanal pull-through procedure for Hirschprung's disease. *Pediatr. Surg. Int.* 2010; 26:1101-1105.

[10] Quinn, F. M., Surana, R., Puri, P. The influence of trisomy 21 on outcome in children with Hirschprung's disease. *J. Pediatr. Surg.* 1994; 29: 781-783.

[11] Austin, K. M. The pathogenesis of Hirschprung's disease-associated enterocolitis. *Semin. Pediatr. Surg.* 2012; 21(4): 319-327.

[12] Elhalaby, E. A. Coran, et al. Enterocolitis associated with Hirschprung's disease: a clinical-radiological characterization based on 168 patients. *J. Pediatr. Surg.* 1995; 30(1): 76-83.

[13] Millar, A. J., Rode, H., Cywes, S. Malrotation and volvulus in infancy and childhood. *Semin. Pediatr. Surg.* 2003; 12: 229-236.

[14] Pickhardt, P. J., Bhalla, S. Intestinal malrotation in adolescents and adults: Spectrum of clinical and imaging features. *AJR Am. J. Roetgenol.* 2002; 179: 1429-1435.

[15] Lake, A. M., Whitington, P. F., Hamilton, S. R. Dietary protein-induced colitis in breast-fed infants. *J. Pediatr.* 1982; 101:906-910.

[16] Pumberger, W., Pomberger, G., Geissler, W. Proctocolitis in breast fed infants: a contribution to differential diagnosis of hematochezia in early childhood. *Postgrad. Med. J.* 2001; 77:252-254.

[17] Anveden, H. L., Finkel, Y., Sandstedt, B., Karpe, B. Proctocolitis in exclusively breast-fed infants. *Eur. J. Pediatr.* 1996; 15:464-467.

[18] Vanderhoof, J. A., Murray, N. D., Kaufman, S. S., et al. Intolerance to protein hydrolysate infant formulas: an underecognized cause of gastrointestinal symptoms in infants. *J. Pediatr.* 1997; 131:741-744.

[19] Høst, A., Jacobsen, H. P., Halken, S., Holmenlund, D. The natural history of cow's milk protein allergy/intolerance. *Eur. J. Clin. Nutr.* 1995; 49 (Suppl.): S13-S18.

[20] Eshel, G., Barr, J., Heyman, E., et al. Intussusception: a 9 year survey (1986-1995). *J. Pediatr. Gastroenterol. Nutr.* 1997; 24: 253-256.

[21] Fischer, T. K., Birhrmann, K., Perch, M., et al. Intussusception in early childhood: a cohort study of 1.7 milion children. *Pediatrics* 2004; 114: 782-5.

[22] Huppertz, H., Soriano-Gabarrò, M., Grimmprel, E., Franco, E., et al., Intussusception Among Young Children in Europe. *Pediatr. Infect. Dis. J.* 2006; 25: S22-S29.

[23] Limas, C., Konstantinos, S., Anagnostoulis, S. Axial torsion and gangrene of a giant Meckel's diverticulum. 2006. *J. Gastrointest. Liver Dis.* 15: 67-68.

[24] Sharma, R., Jain, V. Emergency surgery for Meckel's diverticulum. *World J. Emerg. Surg.* 2008; 3:27.

[25] Giusti, S., Iacconi, C., Giusti, P., Minuto, M., Caramella, D., Bartolozzi, C. Ileal invaginated Meckel's diverticulum: Imaging diagnosis. *Eur. Radiol.* 2004; 14: 2368-2371.

[26] Mayer, C. L., Leibowitz, C. S., Kurosawa, S., Stearns-Kurosawa, D. J. Shiga Toxins and the Pathophysiology of Hemolytic Uremic Syndrome in Humans and Animals. *Toxins* 2012; 4: 1261-1287.

[27] Saulsbury, F. T. Henoch-SchÖnlein purpura in children. Report of 100 patients and review of the literature. *Medicine* 1999; 78(6): 395-409.

[28] Trapani, S., Micheli, A., Grisolia, F., Resti, M., Chiappini, E., Falcini, F., De Martino, M. Henoch-SchÖnlein purpura in childhood: epideimological and clinical analysis of 150 cases over a 5-year period and review of literature. *Semin. Arthr. Rheum.* 2005; 35(3): 143-153.

[29] Ebert, E. C. Gastrointestinal Manifestations of Henoch SchÖnlein Purpura. *Dig. Dis. Sci.* 2008; 53: 2011-2019.

[30] Chang, W. L., Yang, Y. H., Lin, Y. T., Chiang, B. L. Gastrointestinal manifestations in Henoch-SchÖnlein purpura: a review of 261 patients. *Acta Pediatr.* 2004; 93 (11): 1427-1431.

[31] Schwab, J., Benya, E., Lin, R., Majd, K. Contrast enema in children with Henoch-SchÖnlein purpura. *J. Pediatr. Surg.* 2005; 40: 1221-1223.

[32] Kokkonen, J., Kartutten, T. J. Lymphonodular hyperplasia as a sign of food allergy in children. *J. Ped. Gastroenterol. Nutr.* 1999; 29(1): 57-62.

[33] Kaplan, B., Benson, J., Rothstein, F. Lymphonodular hyperplasia of the colon as a pathologic finding in children with lower gastrointestinal bleeding. *J. Ped. Gastroenterol. Nutr.* 1984; 3(5): 704-8.

[34] Iacono, G., Ravelli, A., Di Prima, L., et al. Colonic lymphoid nodular hyperplasia in children: relationship to food hypersensitivity. *Clin. Gastroenterol. Hepatol.* 2007; 5(3): 361-6.

[35] Kuo, H. C., Lee, H. C., Shin, C. H., Sheu, J. C., Chang, P. Y., Wang, N. L. Clinical spectrum of alimentary tract duplication in children. *Acta Pediatr. Taiwan* 2004; 45: 85-8.

[36] Karnak, I., Ocal, T., Senocak, M. E., Tanyel, F. C., et al. Alimentary tract duplications in children: Report of 26 years' experience. *Turk. J. Pediatr.* 2000; 42: 118-25.

[37] Pfeiffer, M. L., DuPont, H. L., Ochoa, T. J. The patient with acute dysentery-A systematic review. *Journal of infection* 2012; 64: 374-386.

[38] Chao, H. C., Chen, C. C., Chen, S. Y., Chiu, C. H. Bacterial enteric infections in children: etiology, clinical manifestations and antimicrobial therapy. *Exp. Rev. Inti. Infect. Ther.* 2006; 4(4): 629-38.

[39] Marcus, R. New information about pediatric foodborne infection. The view from FoodNet. *Curr. Opin. Pediatr.* 2008; 20(1): 79-84.

[40] Erdman, S. H., Barnard, J. A. Gastrointestinal polyps and polyposis syndrome in children. *Current opinion in Pediatrics* 2002; 14: 576-582.

[41] Desai, D. C., Neale, K. F., Talbot, I. C., et al. Juvenile polyposis. *Br. J. Surg.* 1995; 82: 14-7.

[42] Hoffenberg, E. J., Sauaia, A., Malttzam, T., et al. Symptomatic colonic polyps in childhood: not so benign. *J. Pediatr. Gastroenterol. Nutr.* 1999; 28: 175-81.

[43] Beggs, A. D., Latchford, A. R., Vasen, H. F. A., Moslein, G., Alonso, A., et al. Peutz-Jeghers syndrome: a systemic review and recommendations for management. *Gut* 2010; 59: 975-986.

[44] Giardello, F. M., Welsh, S. B., Hamilton, S. R., et al. Increased risk of cancer in Peutz Jeghers syndrome. *N. Engl. J. Med.* 1987, 316: 1511-1514.

[45] Benchimol, E. I., Fortinsky, K. J., Gozdyra, P., Heuvel, M. V. D., Limbergen, J. V., and Griffiths, A. M. Epidemiology of Pediatric Inflammatory Bowel Disease: A Systematic Review of International Trends. *Inflamm. Bowel Dis.* 2011; 17: 423-439.

[46] Inflammatory Bowel Disease in Children and Adolescents: Recommendations for Diagnosis-The Porto Criteria. ESPGHAN IBD Working Group. *J. Pediatr. Gastroenterol. Nutr.* 2005; 41: 1-7.

[47] de la Torre Mondragon, L., Vargas Gomez, M. A., Mora Tiscarreno, M. A., Ramirez Mayans, J. Angiodysplasia of the colon in children. *J. Pediatr. Surg.* 1995; 30: 72-5.

[48] Ponce González, J. F., Sánchez Gil, J. M., Leòn Dueñas, E., Rodriguez, A. Angiodysplasia of the terminal ileum. *Rev. Esp. Enferm. Apar. Dig.* 1989; 75: 179-84.

[49] Chuang, F. J., Lin, J. S., Yeung, C. Y., Chan, W. T., Jiang, C. B., Lee, H. C. Intestinal Angiodysplasia: An Uncommon Cause of Gastrointestinal Bleeding in Children. *Pediatrics and Neonatology* 2011; 52, 214-218.

[50] Junquera, F., Quiroga, S., Saperas, E., et al. Accuracy of helical computed tomographic angiography for the diagnosis of colonic angiodysplasia. *Gastroenterology* 2000; 119: 293-9.

[51] Chua, A. E., Ridley, L. J. Diagnostic accuracy of CT angiography in acute gastrointestinal bleeding. *J. Med. Imaging Radiat. Oncol.* 2008; 52: 333-8.

[52] De la Rubia, L., Ruiz Villespesa, A., Cebrero, M., Garcia de Frias, E. Solitary rectal ulcer syndrome in a child. *J. Pediatr.* 1993; 122: 733-736.

[53] Martin de Carpi, J., Vilar, P., Varea, V. Solitary rectal ulcer syndrome in childhood: a rare, benign, and probably misdiagnosed cause of rectal bleeding. Report of three cases. *Dis. Colon Rectum.* 2007; 50: 534-539.

[54] Ertem, D., Acar, Y., Karaa, E. K., Pehlivanoglu, E. A rare and Often Unrecognized Cause of Hematochezia and Tenesmus in Childhood: Solitary Rectal Ulcer Syndrome. *Pediatrics* 2002; 110: e79.

[55] Dehghani, S. M., Malekpour, A., Haghighat, M. Solitary rectal ulcer syndrome in children: A literature review. *World J. Gastroenterol.* 2012; 18(45): 6541-6545.

[56] Suresh, N., Ganesh, R., Sathiyasekaran, M. Solitary rectal ulcer syndrome: a case series. *Indian Pediatr.* 2010; 47: 1059-1061.

[57] Shcherbina, A., Cooley, J., Lutskiy, M. I., Benarafa, C., Gilbert, G. E., Remold-O'Donnell, E. WASP plays a novel role in regulating platelet responses dependent on alphaIIbbeta3 integrin outsidein signalling. *Br. J. Hematol*. 2010; 148(3): 416-427.

[58] Notarangelo, L. D. In Wiskott-Aldrich syndrome, platelet count matters. *Blood*. 2013; 121(9): 1484-1485.

[59] Nurden, A. T. Glanzmann thrombasthenia. *Orphanet Journal of Rare Disease*. 2006; 1:10: 1-8.

[60] Makris, M. Gastrointestinal bleeding in von Willebrand disease. *Thrombosis Research*. 2006.

[61] Zimmerman, B., Valentino, L. A. Hemophilia: in review. *Pediatr. Rev.* 2013;34(7): 289-94.

[62] Binesh Balachandran and Sunit Singhi. Emergency Management of Lower Gastrointestinal Bleed in Children. *Indian J. Pediatr.* 2013; 80 (3): 219-225.

[63] Squires, Jr R. H. Gastrointestinal bleeding. *Pediatr. Rev.* 1999; 20: 95-101.

[64] Currie, G. M., Kiat, H., Wheat, J. M. Scintigraphic evaluation of acute lower gastrointestinal hemorrhage: current status and future directions. *J. Clin. Gastroenterol*. 2010; 45: 92-9.

In: Clotting Disorders
Editor: Jeffrey L. Wilson

ISBN: 978-1-63482-830-7

Chapter 3

Coagulopathy and Head Trauma

Martin Benčo, MD, PhD
Clinic of Neurosurgery, Jessenius Faculty of Medicine and
University Hospital Martin, Martin, Slovakia

Abstract

Head trauma, a common neurosurgical emergency, is associated with high mortality and morbidity rates. Coagulation disorders, which may be present in head trauma, are associated with worse outcome and increased mortality. There are two major groups of coagulation disorders with essential impact on the outcome after head trauma, which are anticoagulant and antiplatelet therapy and coagulopathy following traumatic brain injury. The first type, with increased occurrence, is caused by the increased use of anticoagulant and antiplatelet treatment in population for cardiovascular diseases. The second type, which may be present in approximately 30-40 % of traumatic brain injury patients, is coagulation disorder following traumatic brain injury. It is characterised by the release of tissue factor and activation of pro-coagulant factors, resulting in complex thrombin formation and conversion of fibrinogen to fibrin. Both types of coagulopathy increase the risk of poor outcome and death among patients with brain trauma.

If the intracranial pressure increases and incranial hypertension occurs, emergency neurosurgical intervention is necessary. Coagulation disorder is a relative contraindication for surgery. On the other hand, surgery leads to consumption of pro-coagulant factors, which may aggravate pre-existing coagulopathy.

This chapter reviews pathogenesis, risk factors and treatment strategy of coagulopathy in patients with craniocerebral injury.

Keywords: Coagulopathy, head trauma

Introduction

Trauma still remains the leading cause of a disability and death in the population younger than 44 years. Worldwide, 15 % of all deaths is a result of an injury, and despite all effort of resuscitation, trauma surgery, and critical care this is expected to rise to almost 20% in the next 15 years. Hemorrhage is the leading mechanism that is responsible for death during the first 24 to 48 hours after trauma. Control of hemorrhage, restoration of circulatory homeostasis and prevention of shock create the basis of the early therapeutic approach to the patient after trauma [1,2].

Head trauma, a common neurosurgical emergency, is associated with high mortality and morbidity rates. One of the most important prognostic factor of the head trauma outcome is coagulopathy [3]. In patients with severe head injury with coagulopathy the mortality was found to be four times higher than in those with head injury, but without any coagulopathy [4]. It has been also found that traumatic brain injury lead to trauma-associated coagulopathy more common than any other trauma. Among injury types, coagulopathy in traumatic brain injury is more common in patients with penetrating injury, probably due to more severe devastation to cerebral tissue and disruption of the barrier between blood and neural tissue [5].

The link between coagulopathy and head trauma is bidirectional. On one hand, the coagulopathy may be present before the head trauma. This is caused by the increased use of anticoagulant and antiplatelet treatment in population for cardiovascular diseases. On other hand, head trauma itself could lead to coagulopathy.

Goodnight *et al.* first describe that tissue thromboplastin, which is present in brain, may be released into the circulation due to trauma, resulting in overactivation of clotting factors. Depletion of coagulation proteins, result of uncontrolled activation of clotting factors may lead to disseminated intravascular coagulopathy (DIC). DIC is characterized by intravascular coagulation, systemic coagulopathy and hemorrhage as a result of the clotting factors consumption [1].

It has been found, that the cause of trauma-associated coagulopathy is multifactorial. Not only consumption and dilution of coagulation factors and platelets but also dysfunctions of coagulation system and platelets, and finally, an increase level in fibrinolysis. This may cause worsening in physiology of injured patients, and create basis for vicious cycle of coagulopathy, hypothermia, and acidosis, a triad which is referred as a lethal triad [6-10].

But, it is still unclear whether it is the development of coagulopathy or the severity of head injury, which predicts the poor outcome for patients after traumatic brain injury.

Anticoagulant and Antiplatelet Treatment and Traumatic Brain Injury

General Considerations

The timing of surgery is based on the urgency of the surgery that depends on type of injury and nature of procedure that have to be performed. For non-emergencies, it is possible to reverse coagulopathy in longer period, but in case of emergencies, it is not possible to wait.

Warfarin

Warfarin is decreasing blood *coagulation* by inhibition of *vitamin K epoxide reductase*. This enzyme convert *oxidized* vitamin K_1 to its reduced form after it has participated in the *carboxylation* of some blood coagulation proteins, mostly *prothrombin* and *factor VII* [11].

In case of need for a non-emergency surgery, the oral antagonist of warfarin is vitamin K, in case of emergencies antidotum of warfarin is protamine [12].

Heparine

The complex of heparin binds to the *antithrombin* III, enzyme inhibitor, lead to conformational change that results in its activation through an increase in the flexibility of its reactive site loop. The activated *antithrombin* III then inactivates *thrombin* and other proteases that are involved in blood clotting, most remarkably *serine endopeptidase* thromboplastin [13].

In patients on heparin, for non-emergencies surgery partial tromboplastin time should be checked 4-6 hours after the heparin cessation, and for emergencies the antidotum is protamine [12].

While heparin and warfarin could be reliably reversed and the reversion could be measured, the situation is less clear with antiplatelets drugs. The agents, that could be used to reverse antiplatelets drugs are fresh frozen plasma and Despmopressin [12].

Acetylsalicylic Acid

Antiplatelet effect of acetylsalicylic acid is based on inhibition of the production of thromboxane, which in normal circumstances binds platelet molecules together to create a plot over interrupted wall of blood vessels [14].

Aggrenox® [acetylsalicylic acid + dipyridamole]

Except of the effect of acetylsalicylic acid, dipyridamole inhibits the phosphodiesterase enzymes that break down cyclic adenosine monophosphate and cyclic guanosine monophosphate. This lead to blocking the platelet response to Adenosine diphosphate. Under the normal conditions, small and disk-shape platelets are circulating in the blood without interaction with each other. Adenosine diphosphate is stored inside the blood platelets in dense bodies and is released during platelet activation. Adenosine diphosphate interacts with a family of specific receptors found on platelets which leads to platelet activation [15].

Plavix® [clopidogrel]

Clopidogrel is irreversibly inhibiting a specific receptor on platelets called $P2Y_{12}$. This receptor is an adenosine diphosphate chemoreceptor on *platelet* cell membranes, which start platelet aggregation.

Platelets should be given, but effect persist for up to a couple of days after last dose of Plavix. In case of continuing bleeding after Plavix discontinuing, next option could trombocyte concentrate or recombinant activated coagulation factor VII - even the defect of coagulation is in platelet, factor VII works through a mechanism not mediated by protein clotting. This treatment is very expensive and must be balanced between the price and repeat operation, prolonged hospital stay and additional morbidity [14].

Pathophysiology of a Traumatic Brain Injury and Trauma-Associated Coagulopathy

The first step of a coagulation cascade starts when platelets are in contact with an subendothelial tissue that have been exposed by vascular injury, that lead to creation of a platelet-rich wedge which is afterwards sustained by fibrin net originate from activation of coagulation cascade and thrombin generation [16]. The changes of platelet functions after traumatic brain injury (TBI) are unclear, but documented low platelet counts in patients without significant blood loss and platelet aggregation suggests, that TBI may lead to platelet hyperactivity. The finding of intravascular microthrombosis in TBI patients also support the presence of platelet hyperactivity [17,18]. Platelet activation and trombi formation in the vessels of brain, but also lungs, was verified in animal model and correlate with clinical finding in patients after TBI. These microthrombi are in brain predominantly detected in the peri-contusion cortex, and are mainly composed of platelets, fibrin and von Willebrand factor [19].

The pathogenesis of platelets hyperactivation is multifactorial. The particularly important role probably plays platelet activating factor (PAF, 1-O-hexadecyl-2-acetyl-sn-glycero-3-phosphocholine). PAF was first described as a molecule that leads to aggregation and serotonin release from platelets in rabbits [20,21], but aftrewards it was identified, that PAF could be synthesized and secreted in many other cells through induced pathways[22]. PAF is acting on target cells through a G-protein-coupled seven transmembrane receptor[22]. The human platelets have two different types of PAF receptors: one with a high affinity and the other with a low affinity. PAF initiates activation of protein kinase C in platelets after binding to the high-affinity receptor [22]. The neural tissue of the brain and spinal cord contain more amount of PAF than other tissues [23] and could be released during ischemia [24].

In addition to a role of PAF during TBI-associated coagulopathy, which is still unclear, it also contributes to the hypoxia-induced disruption of the blood brain barrier, potentially resulting in vicious circle of another PAF release to the systemic circulation [25]. But, on other hand, the use of the drug, that are blocking platelets aggregation did not improve clinical outcome of TBI patients [26]. This lead to the crucial question, which is how to pharmacologically decrease platelets hyperagregability and thus, to improve clinical outcomes of TBI without increasing the risk for intracranial bleeding and its clinical consequences.

Also, another component found in brain microtrombi after TBI, von Willebrand factor, seems to play important role in trauma-associated coagulopathy [19]. VWF, marker for endothelial injury, mediates the initial fixation of platelets to disrupted endothelium or subendothelial matrix at the place of vascular injury [27]. VWF is completely synthesized in endothelial cells and platelets, where is also stored in ultra-large and prothrombotic forms . The stored VWF is released upon stimulation of endothelial cells and platelets [28]. These prothrombotic VWF multimers could be divided by the zinc metalloprotease ADAMTS-13 (a disintegrin and metalloprotease with thrombospondin type 1 repeats) into smaller forms, that are active in hemostasis, but are not prothrombotic. In the absence of this proteolytic activity, VWF multimers form strings that are binding platelets and leukocytes to endothelium. This may lead to thrombi formation and thromboembolism [29,30].

Even if there is no evidence of role of VWF in TBI-associated coagulopathy, there are several suggestions of this possibility. During TBI, the secretion of VWF is notably increased, which is creating pro-trombotic status, and also the activity of ADAMTS-13 is during TBI decreased. On other hand, endothelial cells in cerebral vessels, especially those with small diameter, that are more prone to injury, are synthesizing more VWF than endothelial cells of other organs and VWF and platelets are the main component of microtrombi, that have been found in neural tissue after TBI on animal model [19].

In addition to platelets role in initial clots formation, their also create a surface to initiate extrinsic coagulation pathway. Two key components of extrinsic coagulation pathway, which are tissue factor and phosphatidylserine, are abundantly expressed in neural tissue [19].

Tissue factor , lipoprotein of 263 amino acids , of which the brain tissue is a rich source, is express in endothelial cells, but only after induction by stimulating factors such as injury and inflammation [31,32]. In response to injury, endothelial cells are dropping of a fragments of membrane and are creating an microparticles [33, 34]. They are rich in lipid microdomains where adhesion receptors and tissue factor are highly concentrated [35]. Further, neural cells are highly sensitive to apoptosis and are rapidly producing tissue factor rich neural microparticles [36].

Thus, there are two main reasons for why tissue factor-bearing microparticles may lead to procoagulant activity in neural tissue. On one hand, these microparticles may bring more amount of tissue factor to platelets in neural tissue, what is an explicit mechanism for strengthen of coagulopathy. On other hand microparticles may fuse with other cells, and the coagulation process may be disseminated to other cells, that are normally not involved coagulation cascade, such as neurons [37]. Finally, the fusion of microparticles and target cells also may allow to occur specific cell to cell interactions [between neural cells and platelets or white blood cells], which is physiologically difficult or not possible [19].

Another group of molecules critical for initiating and propagating coagulation is anionic phospholipids. Anionic phospholipids serves as a catalyst that links platelet activation to thrombin generation by providing a highly negatively charged surface and by binding to discrete and specific sites on prothrombin, factor Xa, and factor Va [38]. TBI my lead to discharge of a large amount of phospholipids, which promotes thrombin generation [38,39]. Despite the suggestion, the role of brain phospholipids in the development of TBI-associated coagulopathy remains unknown.

Prognostic Factors Predicting Outcome after TBI

The prognostic factors predicting outcome after TBI have been widely studied. The variables, that could predict unfavourable outcome could be divided into clinical, laboratory and neuroimaging variables. Neuroimaging variables that have been found to be associated with poor outcome are signs of diffuse axonal injury and compression of basal cisterns. The presence and size of the SDH or EDH, the presence, size, and location of the contusion, combined injury, and midline shift were not significantly associated with an unfavorable outcome. Seven of the nine patients with a contusion larger than 60 cm^3 regained good function [40,41]. The clinical variables, that were identified as an independent prognostic factor of an unfavorable outcome TBI caused by motorcycle accident. If the patients were injured during the motorcycle accidents they were more likely to have an poor outcome compared to other types of injury. On other hand gender and presence of an acute seizure did not predict poor outcome [40,41]. The impact of age on the prognosis of TBI is still not clear, some authors have noted varied age thresholds for poor prognosis [41,42,43]. This threshold varied in different studies and have been noted from 35 to 50 years, respectively some authors [44, 45] noted, that 60 years could be the critical threshold for the poor outcome after TBI [46, 47]. The impact of age on outcome is probably due to the decreased capacity of adult brain for recovery as it ages, due to decreasing number of functioning neurons and greater exposure to subclinical insults. The laboratory variables, that were identified as a significant predictors of poor outcome after TBI were hypoxia, the unstable blood pressure, pulse, oxygen saturation and coagulopathy [48, 49, 50, 51].

Trauma-Associated Coagulopathy and Traumatic Brain Injury

In the literature the incidence of coagulopathy in TBI varies considerably among different studies. The reported incidence ranges between 10 and 97% [52,53,54,55,56]. This wide differences in incidence of coagulopathy in TBI through various studies could be the result of different criteria, that have been used by different authors to definition of coagulopathy. In this studies, there were variable inclusion criteria, and variable degree of severity of the head trauma. So far, there is no standard definition for coagulopathy in TBI. The risk factors, that have been found to be independent risk factors associated developing coagulopathy in patients with isolated TBI were Glasgow Coma Scale (GCS≤8) or a high Injury Severity Score (ISS≥16), acidosis, hypotension on admission, and the presence of cerebral edema, subarachnoid hemorrhage, and midline shift [12]. Some other studies shown, that effaced cistern in the CT have association with development of coagulopathy, but contusion, hemorrhage, midline shift, intracranial fracture, effaced cisterns and diffuse axonal injury were identified not to be the risk factor for coagulopathy development [51]. The TBI patients with coagulopathy were found to have significantly increased PT, INR, APTT and thrombin time at the time of admission [51].

As some authors have shown, the children might be in higher risk of both, TBI and also of developing of coagulopathy after TBI, compared to adults [57, 58]. There are several reasons of this possibility. It have been found, that in car accident, that are one of the most common reason of TBI of children, the head is the body part most frequently and most seriously involved. Also, the frequency of TBI was found to be much greater than either adolescents or adults. The reasons for this greater frequency of head injury in children can be the result of the fact, that child's head is proportionately larger and heavier and neck supporting structures are weaker, than in the adult. On other hand, children the head is also relatively soft, pliable, and elastic bones of the cranial vault, and the fontanelles that make the head of the child less secure against to trauma impact. And, also, infant head shape also differs significantly from that of the adult. In the infant the cranium is much more elongate and bulbous, with large frontal and parietal prominences due to the massive size of the frontal lobe of the brain. And, finally, the child's head is proportionately larger than in the adult [57, 59, 60].

The Treatment of TBI Associated Coagulopathy

Human recombinant activated factor-VII (rFVIIa) has been successfully used in the treatment of spontaneous intracerebral hemorrhage. Thus, several authors focused on potential effect of rFVIIa on trauma associated coagulopathy. In animal model, the use of rFVIIa reduced expansion of traumatic contusion and provide protection to axons and hippocampal neurons. This animal model shows the potential of rFVIIa to be the clinically successful medical therapy for TBI [61]. Even if there were several worldwide trial of FVIIa in trauma patients, focused on the therapy of hemorrhagic shock, this studies excludes patients with severe TBI. So, there was urgent need to study this trauma population [62]. Two systematic studies were compared by Perel [63,64,65]. Both evaluated the effects of recombinant factor VIIa (rFVIIa). The earlier trial was a post hoc analysis of traumatic brain injury patients from a randomised controlled trial of rFVIIa in blunt trauma patients [63]. The later one, focused on the effects of rFVIIa in TBI patients with evidence of intracerebral bleeding on CT scan obtained within six hours of the injury [64]. The comparison of these studies showed, that there is no reliable evidence that the use of rFVIIa is effective in reducing mortality or disability in patients with TBI [65]. And, finally, the CRASH-II study showed, that there is no no evidence of the effect of tranexamic acid on death due to bleeding varied by systolic blood pressure, Glasgow coma score, or type of injury [66].

Even if the results of some previous studies did not show the benefit of use of rFVIIa and tranexamic acid on outcome of trauma patients, in case of need for a urgent surgery this could be the only way, how to normalise coagulation and perform surgery [63,64,65,66]. There is still need for further evaluation of trauma-associated coagulopathy, because its development stay important factor of poor outcome in TBI patients, and it is still unclear if the treatment, that allows performing surgery may improve the outcome or not.

References

[1] Gruen RL, Brohi K, Schreiber M, Balogh ZJ, Pitt V, Narayan M, Maier RV. Haemorrhage control in severely injured patients. *Lancet.* 2012 Sep; 380(9847):1099-108.

[2] Maegele M, Spinella PC, Schöchl H. The acute coagulopathy of trauma: mechanisms and tools for risk stratification. *Shock.* 2012; 38(5):450-8.

[3] Lapointe LA, Von Rueden KT. Coagulopathies in trauma patients. *AACN Clin. Issues.* 2002; 13(2):192-203.

[4] Bellamy RF, Maningas PA, Vayer JS. Epidemiology of trauma: military experience. *Ann. Emerg. Med.* 1986; 15(12):1384-8.

[5] Harhangi BS, Kompanje EJ, Leebeek FW, Maas AI. Coagulation disorders after traumatic brain injury. *Acta Neurochir.* (Wien). 2008; 150(2):165-75.

[6] Goodnight SH, Kenoyer G, Rapaport SI, Patch MJ, Lee JA, Kurze T. Defibrination after brain-tissue destruction: A serious complication of head injury. *N. Engl. J. Med.* 1974; 290(19):1043-7.

[7] Wafaisade A, Wutzler S, Lefering R, Tjardes T, Banerjee M, Paffrath T, Bouillon B,Maegele M. Drivers of acute coagulopathy after severe trauma: a multivariate analysis of 1987 patients. Emerg. *Med. J.* 2010;27:934–939.

[8] Maani CV, DeSocio PA, Holcomb JB. Coagulopathy in trauma patients: what are the main influence factors? *Curr. Opin. Anaesthesiol.* 2009;22:255–260.

[9] Mitra B, Cameron PA, Mori A, Maini A, Fitzgerald M, Paul E, Street A. Early prediction of acute traumatic coagulopathy. *Resuscitation.* 2011;82:1208–1213.

[10] Mitra B, Tullio F, Cameron PA, Fitzgerald M. Trauma patients with the 'triad of death'. *Emerg. Med. J.*2012;29:622–625.

[11] Ansell J, Hirsh J, Hylek E, et al. (2008). Pharmacology and management of the vitamin K antagonists: American College of Chest Physicians evidence-based clinical practice guidelines (8th Edition)". Chest 133 (6 Suppl).2008;: 160S–198S.

[12] Greenberg MS (ed.). Handbook of neurosurgery 7th edition ed. Thieme Publishers, New York, 2010, pp 34-43.

[13] Björk I, Lindahl U. Mechanism of the anticoagulant action of heparin. *Mol. Cell Biochem.* 1982; 48(3):161-82.

[14] Enomoto Y, Yoshimura S. Antiplatelet Therapy for Carotid Artery Stenting. *Interv. Neurol.* 2013; 1(3-4): 151–163. 14.

[15] Murugappa S, Kunapuli SP. The role of ADP receptors in platelet function. *Front. Biosci.* 2006;11: 1977–86.

[16] Zhang J, Jiang R, Liu L, Watkins T, Zhang F, Dong JF. Traumatic brain injury-associated coagulopathy. *J. Neurotrauma.* 2012; 29 (17):2597-605.

[17] Kaufman HH, Hui KS, Mattson JC, Borit A, Childs TL, Hoots WK, Bernstein DP, Makela ME, Wagner KA, Kahan BD, et al. Clinicopathological correlations of disseminated intravascular coagulation in patients with head injury. *Neurosurgery.* 1984;15:34–42.

[18] Stein SC, Graham DI, Chen XH, Smith DH. Association between intravascular microthrombosis and cerebral ischemia in traumatic brain injury. *Neurosurgery.* 2004;54:687–691.

[19] Lu D, Mahmood A, Goussev A, Qu C, Zhang ZG, Chopp M. Delayed thrombosis after traumatic brain injury in rats. *J. Neurotrauma.* 2004;21:1756–1766.

[20] Henson PM. Release of vasoactive amines from rabbit platelets induced by sensitized mononuclear leukocytes and antigen. *J. Exp. Med.* 1970;131:287–30.

[21] Benveniste J, Henson PM, Cochrane CG. Leukocyte-dependent histamine release from rabbit platelets. The role of IgE, basophils, and a platelet-activating factor. *J. Exp. Med.* 1972;136:1356–1377.

[22] Chao W, Olson MS. Platelet-activating factor: receptors and signal transduction. *Biochem. J.* 1993;292:617–629.

[23] Kumar R, Harvey SA, Kester M, Hanahan DJ, Olson MS. Production and effects of platelet-activating factor in the rat brain. *Biochim. Biophys. Acta.* 1988;963:375–383.

[24] Nishida K, Markey SP. Platelet-activating factor in brain regions after transient ischemia in gerbils. *Stroke.* 1996;27(3):514-8.

[25] Deng Y, Fang W, Li Y, Cen J, Fang F, Lv P, Gong S, Mao L. Blood-brain barrier breakdown by PAF and protection by XQ-1H due to antagonism of PAF effects. *Eur. J. Pharmacol.* 2009;616:43–47.

[26] Wong DK, Lurie F, Wong LL. The effects of clopidogrel on elderly traumatic brain injured patients. *J. Trauma.* 2008;65:1303–1308.

[27] De Oliveira CO, Reimer AG, Da Rocha AB, Grivicich I, Schneider RF, Roisenberg I, Regner A, Simon D. Plasma von Willebrand factor levels correlate with clinical outcome of severe traumatic brain injury. *J. Neurotrauma.* 2007;24:1331–1338.

[28] Moake JL, Chow TW. Increased von Willebrand factor (vWf) binding to platelets associated with impaired vWf breakdown in thrombotic thrombocytopenic purpura. *J. Clin. Apheresis.* 1998;13:126–132.

[29] Dong JF, Moake JL, Nolasco L, Bernardo A, Arceneaux W, Shrimpton CN, Schade AJ, McIntire LV, Fujikawa K, Lopez J.A. ADAMTS-13 rapidly cleaves newly secreted ultralarge von Willebrand factor multimers on the endothelial surface under flowing conditions. *Blood.* 2002;100:4033–4039.

[30] Spicer EK, Horton R, Bloem L, Bach R, Williams KR, Guha A, Kraus J, Lin TC, Nemerson Y, Konigsberg WH. Isolation of cDNA clones coding for human tissue factor: primary structure of the protein and cDNA. *Proc. Natl. Acad. Sci. USA.* 1987;84:5148–5152.

[31] Bevilacqua MP, Pober JS, Majeau GR, Fiers W, Cotran RS, Gimbrone MA Jr. Recombinant tumor necrosis factor induces procoagulant activity in cultured human vascular endothelium: characterization and comparison with the actions of interleukin 1. *Proc. Natl. Acad. Sci. USA.* 1986;83:4533–4537.

[32] Astrup T. Assay and content of tissue thromboplastin in different organs. Thromb. *Diath. Haemorrh.* 1965;14:401–416.

[33] Siljander P, Farndale RW, Feijge MA, Comfurius P, Kos S, Bevers EM, Heemskerk JW. Platelet adhesion enhances the glycoprotein VI-dependent procoagulant response: involvement of p38 MAP kinase and calpain. Arterioscler. *Thromb. Vasc. Biol.* 2001;21:618–627.

[34] Bode AP, Orton SM, Frye MJ, Udis BJ. Vesiculation of platelets during in vitro aging. *Blood.* 1991;77:887–895.

[35] Biro E, Akkerman JW, Hoek FJ, Gorter G, Pronk LM, Sturk A, Nieuwland R. The phospholipid composition and cholesterol content of platelet-derived microparticles: a comparison with platelet membrane fractions. *J. Thromb. Haemost.* 2005;3:2754–2763.

[36] Bianco F, Pravettoni E, Colombo A, Schenk U, Moller T, Matteoli M, Verderio C. Astrocyte-derived ATP induces vesicle shedding and IL-1 beta release from microglia. *J. Immunol.* 2005;174:7268–7277.

[37] Faille D, El-Assaad F, Mitchell AJ, Alessi MC, Chimini G, Fusai T, Grau GE, Combes V. Endocytosis and intracellular processing of platelet microparticles by brain endothelial cells. *J. Cell Mol. Med.* 2011:10–4934.

[38] Lentz BR. Exposure of platelet membrane phosphatidylserine regulates blood coagulation. *Prog. Lipid Res.* 2003;42:423–438.

[39] Lee SY, Oh MK. Response to: Prediction of Outcome after Traumatic Brain Injury Using Clinical and Neuroimaging Variables: A Methodological Mistake. *J. Clin. Neurol.* 2013;9(3):198.

[40] Lee SY, Kim SS, Kim CH, Park SW, Park JH, Yeo M. Prediction of outcome after traumatic brain injury using clinical and neuroimaging variables. *J. Clin. Neurol.* 2012;8(3):224-9.

[41] Gómez PA, Lobato RD, Boto GR, De la Lama A, González PJ, de la Cruz J. Age and outcome after severe head injury. *Acta Neurochir.* (Wien) 2000;142:373–80.

[42] Bricolo A, Turazzi S, Alexandre A, Rizzuto N. Decerebrate rigidity in acute head injury. *J. Neurosurg.* 1977;47:680–98.

[43] Vollmer DG, Torner JC, Jane JA, Sadovnic B, Charlebois D, Eisenberg HM, et al. Age and outcome following traumatic coma: why do older patients fare worse? *J. Neurosurg.* (suppl) 1991;75:S37–49.

[44] Bricolo A, Turazzi S, Alexandre A, Rizzuto N. Decerebrate rigidity in acute head injury. *J. Neurosurg.* 1977;47:680–98.

[45] Signorini DF, Andrews PJ, Jones PA, Wardlaw JM, Miller JD. Predicting survival using simple clinical variables; a case study in traumatic brain injury. *J. Neurol. Neurosurg. Psychiatry.* 1999;60:20–5.

[46] The Brain Trauma Foundation. The American Association of Neurological Surgeons. The Joint Section on Neurotrauma and Critical Care. *J. Neurotrauma.* 2000;17:555–81.

[47] Heiskanen O, Sipponen P. Prognosis of severe brain injury. *Acta Neurol. Scand.* 1970;46:343–8.

[48] Sharda P, Haspani S, Idris Z.Factors prognosticating the outcome of decompressive craniectomy in severe traumatic brain injury: A Malaysian experience. *Asian J. Neurosurg.* 2014;9(4):203-12.

[49] Gaddam SS, Buell T, Robertson CS. Systemic manifestations of traumatic brain injury. *Handb. Clin. Neurol.* 2015;127:205-18.

[50] Edavettal M, Vellucci A, Rogers FB. Traumatic brain injury is not associated with coagulopathy out of proportion to injury in other body regions. *J. Trauma Acute Care Surg*. 2014;77(5):799.

[51] [51] Chhabra G, Sharma S, Subramanian A, Agrawal D, Sinha S, Mukhopadhyay AK. Coagulopathy as prognostic marker in acute traumatic brain injury. *J. Emerg. Trauma Shock*. 2013; 6(3): 180–185.

[52] Miner ME, Kaufman HH, Graham SH, Haar FH, Gildenberg PL. Disseminated intravascular coagulation fibrinolytic syndrome following head injury in children: Frequency and prognostic implications. *J. Pediatr*. 1982;100:687–91.

[53] Olson JD, Kaufman HH, Moake J, O'Gorman TW, Hoots K, Wagner K, et al. The incidence and significance of hemostatic abnormalities in patients with head injuries. *Neurosurgery*. 1989;24:825–32.

[54] Kearney TJ, Bentt L, Grode M, Lee S, Hiatt JR, Shabot MM. Coagulopathy and catecholamines in severe head injury. *J. Trauma*. 1992;32:608–11.

[55] Cohen MJ, Brohi K, Ganter MT, Manley GT, Mackersie RC, Pittet JF. Early coagulopathy after traumatic brain injury: The role of hypoperfusion and the protein C pathway. *J. Trauma*. 2007;63:1254–61.

[56] Kaufman HH, Hui KS, Mattson JC, Borit A, Childs TL, Hoots WK, et al. Clinicopathological correlations of disseminated intravascular coagulation in patients with head injury. *Neurosurgery*. 1984;15:34–42.

[57] M. Benčo, J. De Riggo, S. Nosáľ, M. Fedor, J. Šutovský, R. Opšenák. A Coagulopathy Following Craniocerebral Injury in Children and Adolescents. *Cesk. Slov. Neurol.* N 2012; 75/108(4): 432-437.

[58] Dhandapani SS, Manju D, Sharma BS, Mahapatra AK. Prognostic significance of age in traumatic brain injury. *J. Neurosci. Rural. Pract.* 2012; 3(2): 131–135.

[59] Donald F. Huelke. An Overview of Anatomical Considerations of Infants and Children in the Adult World of Automobile Safety Design. *Annu. Proc. Assoc. Adv. Automot. Med*. 1998; 42: 93–113.

[60] Agran PF, Winn D. Traumatic Injuries Among Children Using Lap Belts and Lap/Shoulder Belts in Motor Vehicle Collisions. 31st Proc. *Am. Assn. for Auto Med*. 1987:183–307.

[61] Zhang J, Groff RF 4th, Chen XH, Browne KD, Huang J, Schwartz ED, Meaney DF, Johnson VE, Stein SC, Rojkjaer R, Smith DH. Hemostatic and neuroprotective effects of human recombinant activated factor VII therapy after traumatic brain injury in pigs. *Exp. Neurol.* 2008;210(2):645-55.

[62] Richard P Dutton. Factor VII and the brain: time to get this research done! *Crit. Care.* 2007; 11(4): 161.

[63] Kluger Y, Riou B, Rossaint R, Rizoli SB, Boffard KD, Choong PI, Warren B, Tillinger M. Safety of rFVIIa in hemodynamically unstable polytrauma patients with traumatic brain injury: post hoc analysis of 30 patients from a prospective, randomized, placebo-controlled, double-blind clinical trial. *Crit. Care.* 2007; 11(4):R85

[64] Boffard KD, Riou B, Warren B, Choong PI, Rizoli S, Rossaint R, Axelsen M, Kluger Y, NovoSeven Trauma Study Group. Recombinant factor VIIa as adjunctive therapy for bleeding control in severely injured trauma patients: two parallel randomized, placebo-controlled, double-blind clinical trials. J Trauma. 2005; 59(1):8-15.1Department of Neurosurgery, Tianjin Medical University and Tianjin Neurology Institute, Tianjin, China.

[65] Perel P, Roberts I, Shakur H, Thinkhamrop B, Phuenpathom N, Yutthakasemsunt S. Haemostatic drugs for traumatic brain injury. *Cochrane Database Syst. Rev.* 2010; (1): CD007877.

[66] CRASH-2 collaborators, Roberts I, Shakur H, Afolabi A, Brohi K, Coats T, Dewan Y, Gando S, Guyatt G, Hunt BJ, Morales C, Perel P, Prieto-Merino D, Woolley T. The importance of early treatment with tranexamic acid in bleeding trauma patients: an exploratory analysis of the CRASH-2 randomised controlled trial. *Lancet.* 2011;377 (9771): 1096-101, 1101.e1-2.

In: Clotting Disorders
Editor: Jeffrey L. Wilson

ISBN: 978-1-63482-830-7

Chapter 4

Vitamin B_{12} Modulates AM-Coagulation

*Thomas Stief**
Institute of Laboratory Medicine and Pathobiochemistry,
University Hospital Giessen & Marburg, Germany

Abstract

Background: Cobalamin is the hydrophilic vitamin B_{12} of a complicated structure with a central cobalt ion for normal erythropoiesis and nerve function. Vitamin B_{12} can clinically be given as 1000-1500 µg injections. Therefore, this work quantified the changed thrombin generation by altered matrix (AM) thru an increase of plasmatic vitamin B_{12} concentration.

Material and Methods: 40 µl platelet poor citrated plasma of 12 healthy donors were supplemented either with 0-610 µg/l hydroxocobalamin acetate or with 0-610 µg/l cyanocobalamine by repetitive 1+1 dilution on the polystyrene microtiter plate (Brand®781600). The RECA was performed with 10 or 20 min (37°C) coagulation reaction time. The approx. SC200 or approx. IC50 was determined for each individual plasma.

* Correspondence to: PD Dr. med. T. Stief, Central Laboratory, University Hospital, D-35043 Marburg, Germany; email: thstief@t-online.de; Tel. : +49-6421-58 64471; FAX: +49-6421-58 65594.

Results and Discussion: The approx. SC200 on AM-coagulation was 19±14 µg/l (MV±1SD) hydroxocobalamin acetate in 5 of 6 plasmas; one plasma had an approx. IC50 of 8 µg/l. Cyanocobalamin had an approx. SC200 of 101±130 µg/l in 3 of 6 plasmas and an approx. IC50 of 13±14 µg/l in 3 of 6 samples. This means that there are hemostasis differences between hydroxocobalamin acetate and cyanocobalamin. Hydroxocobalamin acetate triggers intrinsic coagulation much more than cyanocobalamin. This might be due to the acetate part of the hydroxocobalamin drug. It could be of pharmacologic interest to substitute acetate in hydroxocobalamin by HCl.

Introduction

Vitamin B_{12} with its 4 cobalamin vitamers adenosyl-, methyl-, cyano-, and hydroxo- is a C_1 transferring with folate cooperating vitamin, necessary for the generation of erythrocytes and for normal nerve function [1-4]. The drug vitamin B_{12} acts against cobalamin deficiency, transcobalamin deficiency, and cyanide poisoning. For the latter indication, a large amount of hydroxocobalamine is given intravenously; cyanide converts hydroxo- in cyano-cobalamine that is excreted in urine.

The daily requirement of vitamin B_{12} is about 3 µg [1]. The normal plasma concentration is about 200-900 ng/l [5].

Vitamin B_{12} is clinically available in 1-1.5 mg amounts per ampoule. Since cobalamin is of such a complicated molecular structure (Fig. 1) injection of cobalamin could induce a blood matrix change, causing altered matrix (AM)-coagulation activation [6,7]; negatively charged or lipophilic molecules fold factor 12 into F12a or pre-kallikrein into kallikrein [8-11]. The best assay to determine even spurious activations of AM-coagulation in plasma is the recalcified coagulation activity assay (RECA) [12].

Vitamin B_{12} in its 4 vitamer forms adenosylcobalamin, methylcobalamin, hydroxocobalamin, and cyanocobalamin (figure 1 upper image) [1]. The hydroxocobalamin·HCl form (figure 1 lower image) [2] has the sum formula $C_{62}H_{89}CoN_{13}O_{15}P \cdot HCl$ (1382.8 Daltons). Vitamin B_{12} is absorbed together with intrinsic factor in the distal half of the ileum. In blood it is transported by transcobalamin.

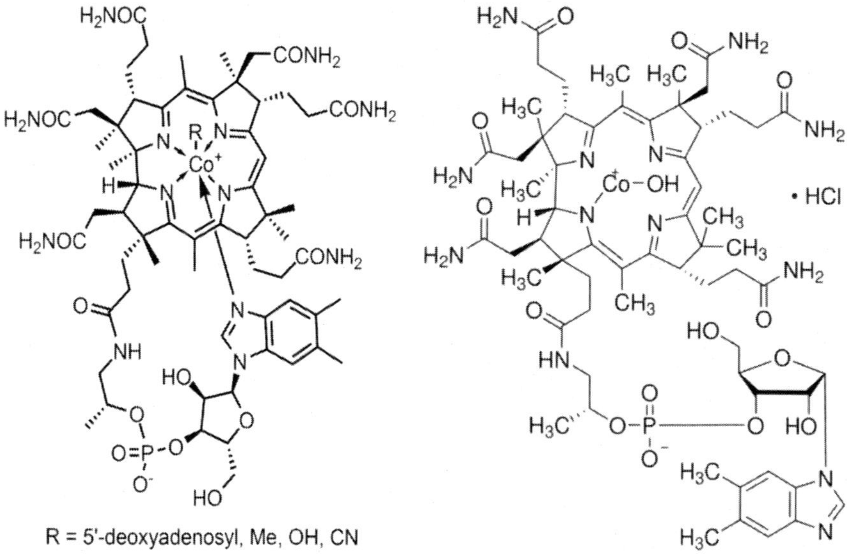

Figure 1. Chemical structure of vitamin B12 (cobalamin) [1]. Vitamin B_{12} (cobalamin; IUPAC name: α-(5,6-dimethylbenzimidazolyl)cobamidcyanide) with a molecular mass of 1355.4 Daltons of its adenosyl-form ($C_{63}H_{88}CoN_{14}O_{14}P$) as the largest and most structurally complicated vitamin cannot be synthesized chemically up to now, the main structure of hydroxo-cobalamin is industrially produced by bacteria. The center of vitamin B_{12} is a corrin ring, i.e. a tetra-pyrrole ring with a central cobalt ion. The corrin ring is similar to the porphyrin ring in heme, chlorophyll, and cytochrome. 4 of the 6 binding sites of the cobalt ion are occupied by the corrin ring, binding site 5 is dimethylbenzimidazole . Binding site 6 (R) is the center of reactivity: there at least 4 vitamers of vitamin B_{12} with R = 5´-deoxyadenosyl (C_5 atom of deoxyribose binding to Co), methyl (Me), OH (hydroxyl), or C≡N (cyano), all of them have vitamin activity. The human body converts a B_{12} vitamer into the natural cofactors a) methyl-cobalamin (MeB_{12}), the cofactor of the enzyme methionine synthetase that converts homocysteine to methionine and 5-methyltetrahydrofolate to tetrahydrofolate or adenosyl-cobalamin and b) adenosyl-cobalamin ($AdoB_{12}$), the cofactor of methylmalonyl coenzyme A mutase (MUT). For food supplements usually the cheap cyano-cobalamin is used, the therefrom released cyanide together with tobacco smoke might damage the nervus opticus. The vitamin is absorbed in complex with "intrinsic factor" of HCl producing parietal cells of the stomach in the distal ileum. In blood it is transported by transcobalamin. The half-life is about 6d (about 1 year in the liver), it is renally eliminated [1].

Material and Methods

40 µl -30°C frozen/23°C thawed platelet poor citrated plasma of 12 healthy donors were supplemented after written informed consent either with 0-609.8 µg/l hydroxocobalamin acetate (Pascoe, Giessen, Germany; 1 ml

ampoules of 1500 μg) or with cyanocobalamin (Jenapharm, Brehna, Germany; 1 ml ampoules of 1000 μg) by repetitive 1+1 dilution on the polystyrene microtiter plate (Brand, Wertheim, Germany; article nr. 781600). The RECA was started with 4 μl 250 mM $CaCl_2$ (Sigma, Deisenhofen, Germany) After 0, 10, or 20 min (37°C) coagulation reaction time (CRT) the RECA was stopped by addition of 80 μl 2.5 M arginine, pH 8.6, 0.16% Triton X 100® (Sigma). After 3 min 20 μl chromogenic thrombin substrate 1 mM HD-CHG-Ala-Arg-pNA (Pentapharm, Basel, Switzerland) in 1.25 M arginine, pH 8.7, were added and the increase in absorbance with time ΔA/t was determined at 405 nm by a microtiter plate photometer with a 1 mA resolution (PHOmo; Autobio-anthos, Krefeld, Germany). The approximate 200% stimulatory concentrations (approx. SC200) or the approximate 50% inhibitory concentrations (approx. IC50) were determined for the individual plasmas at the most sensible thrombin generation curve. Considered were only the thrombin activities in the ascending part of the CRT vs. thrombin activity generation curve.

Results and Discussion

Figures 2-7 demonstrate the results of hydroxocobalamin acetate, figures 8-13 that of cyanocobalamin. The approx. SC200 on AM-coagulation was 19±14 μg/l (MV±1SD) hydroxocobalamin acetate in 5 of 6 plasmas; one plasma had an approx. IC50 of 8 μg/l (Fig. 6). Cyanocobalamin had an approx. SC200 of 101±130 μg/l in 3 of 6 plasmas and an approx. IC50 of 13±14 μg/l in 3 of 6 samples. This means that there are pronounced hemostasis differences between hydroxocobalamin acetate and cyanocobalamin. Hydroxocobalamin acetate triggers intrinsic coagulation more than cyanocobalamin. This might be due to the acetate part of the hydroxocobalamin drug. Acetate triggers intrinsic coagulation with approx. SC200 values in the range of about 10 μM [13]. It could be of pharmacologic interest to substitute acetate in hydroxocobalamin by HCl. Cobalamin injection in hemostasis susceptible patients [14,15] might be accompanied by low-molecular-weight-heparin (LMWH) thrombosis prophylaxis [16].

The question arises why there are plasmas that respond to vitamin B_{12} addition with an IC50 instead of a SC200. Here cobalamin seems to stop AM-coagulation by blocking protein/protein interactions. In certain plasmas cobalamin could attach to certain important proteins of intrinsic coagulation and act as an AM-coagulation interrupter [11]. Clarifying the exact mechanism of AM-coagulation interruption could be of pharmacologic interest.

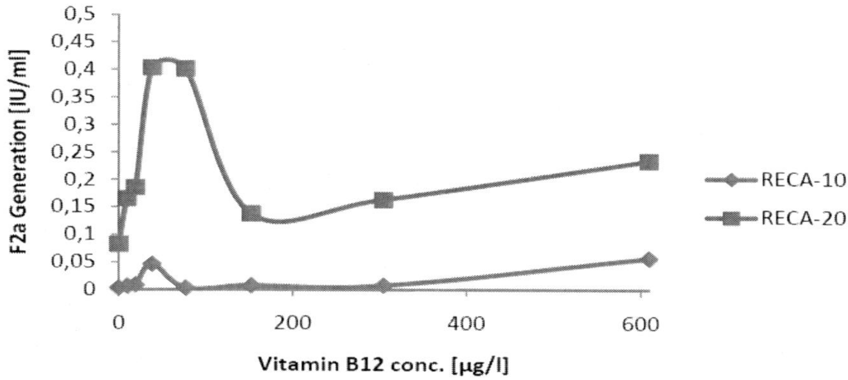

Figure 2. SC200 determination in plasma 1. 40 µl citrated plasma 1, supplemented with 0-610 µg/l hydroxocobalamin acetate, were recalcified and the thrombin generation was stopped after 10 min or 20 min by arginine as described under Methods. The approx. SC200 was 9 µg/l.

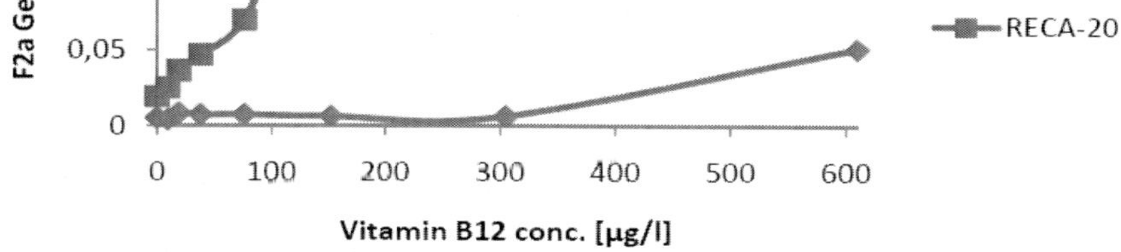

Figure 3. SC200 determination in plasma 2. 40 µl citrated plasma 2, supplemented with 0-610 µg/l hydroxocobalamin acetate, were recalcified and the thrombin generation was stopped after 10 min or 20 min by arginine as described under Methods. The approx. SC200 was 20 µg/l.

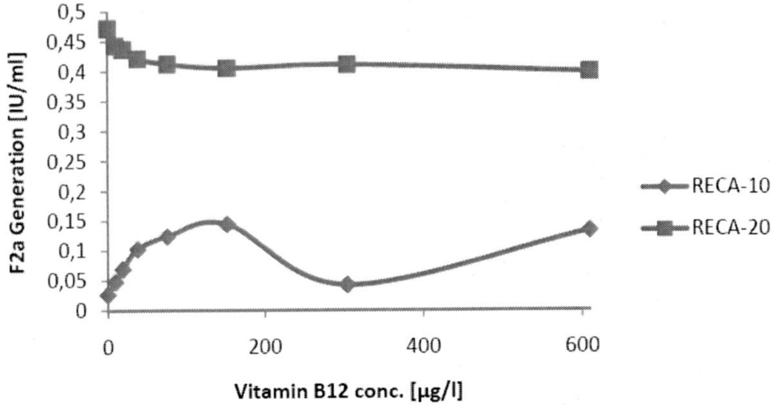

Figure 4. SC200 determination in plasma 3.

40 µl citrated plasma 3, supplemented with 0-610 µg/l hydroxocobalamin acetate, were recalcified and the thrombin generation was stopped after 10 min or 20 min by arginine as described under Methods. The approx. SC200 was 4 µg/l.

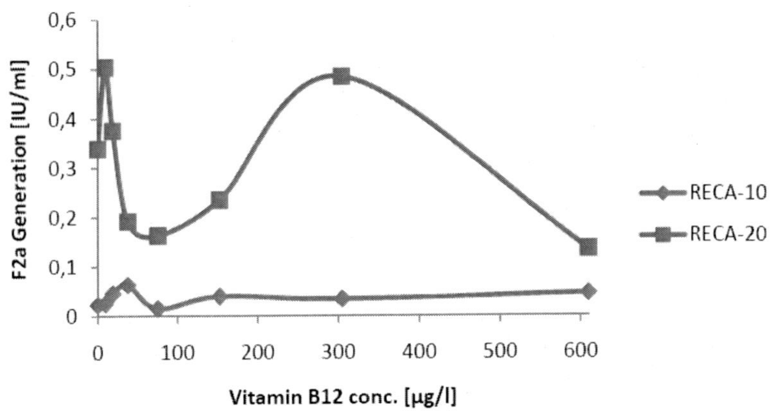

Figure 5. SC200 determination in plasma 4.

40 µl citrated plasma 4, supplemented with 0-610 µg/l hydroxocobalamin acetate, were recalcified and the thrombin generation was stopped after 10 min or 20 min by arginine as described under Methods. The approx. SC200 was 20 µg/l.

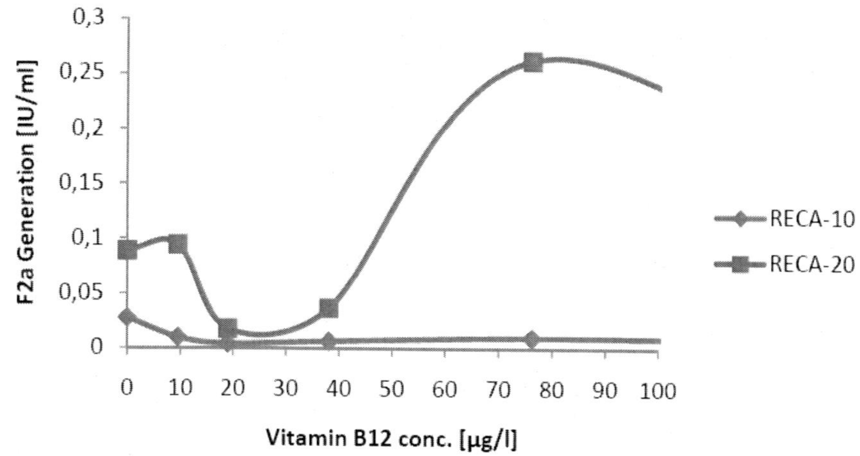

Figure 6. IC50, SC200 determination in plasma 5.

40 µl citrated plasma 5, supplemented with 0-610 µg/l hydroxocobalamin acetate, were recalcified and the thrombin generation was stopped after 10 min or 20 min by arginine as described under Methods. The approx. IC50 was 8 µg/l, the approx. SC200 was 55 µg/l.

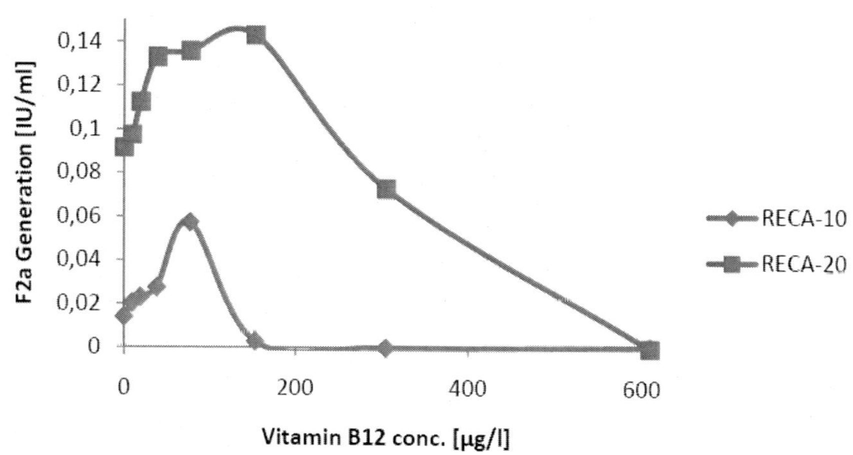

Figure 7. SC200 determination in plasma 6.

40 µl citrated plasma 6, supplemented with 0-610 µg/l hydroxocobalamin acetate, were recalcified and the thrombin generation was stopped after 10 min or 20 min by arginine as described under Methods. The approx. SC200 was 40 µg/l.

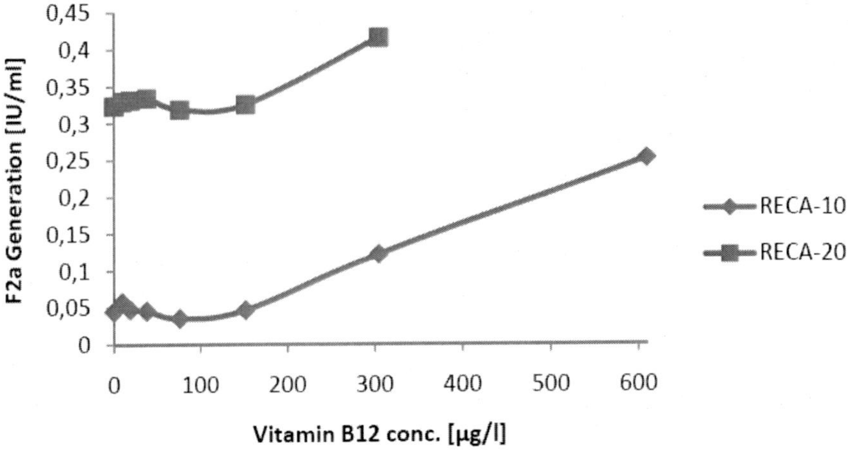

Figure 8. SC200 determination in plasma 7.

40 µl citrated plasma 7, supplemented with 0-610 µg/l cyanocobalamin, were recalcified and the thrombin generation was stopped after 10 min or 20 min by arginine as described under Methods. The approx. SC200 was 250 µg/l.

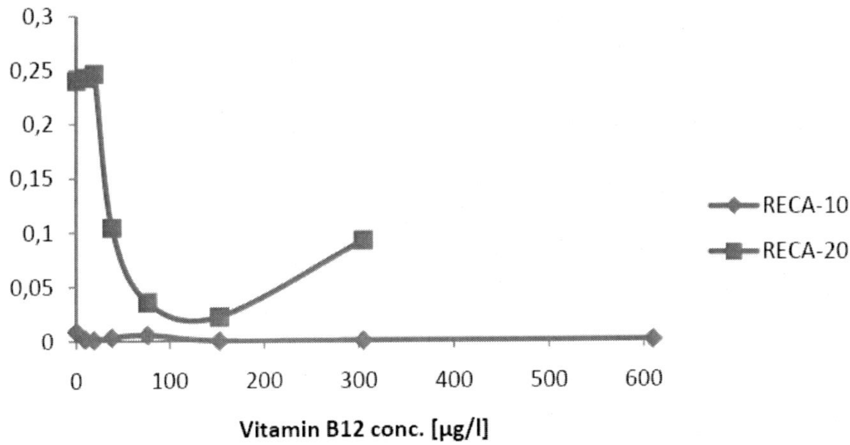

Figure 9. IC50 determination in plasma 8.

40 µl citrated plasma 8, supplemented with 0-610 µg/l cyanocobalamin, were recalcified and the thrombin generation was stopped after 10 min or 20 min by arginine as described under Methods. The approx. IC50 was 30 µg/l.

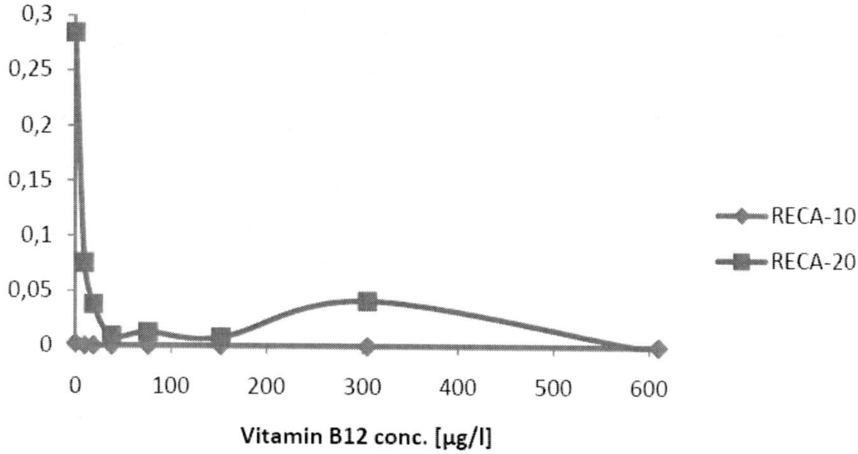

Figure 10. IC50 determination in plasma 9.

40 µl citrated plasma 9, supplemented with 0-610 µg/l cyanocobalamin, were recalcified and the thrombin generation was stopped after 10 min or 20 min by arginine as described under Methods. The approx. IC50 was 5 µg/l.

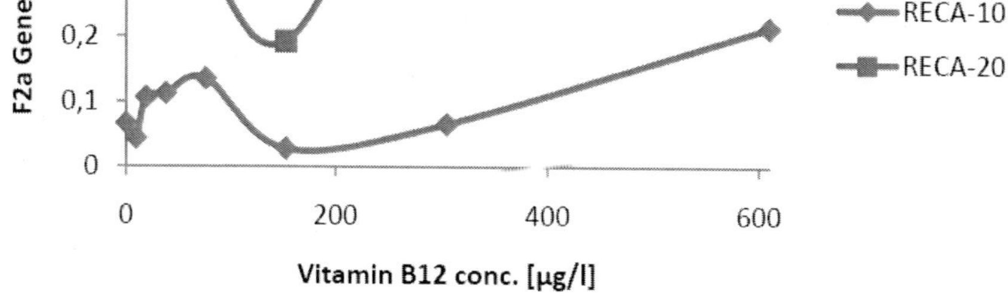

Figure 11. SC200, IC50 determination in plasma 10.

40 µl citrated plasma 10, supplemented with 0-610 µg/l cyanocobalamin, were recalcified and the thrombin generation was stopped after 10 min or 20 min by arginine as described under Methods. The approx. SC200 was 75 µg/l, the approx. IC50 was 130 µg/l.

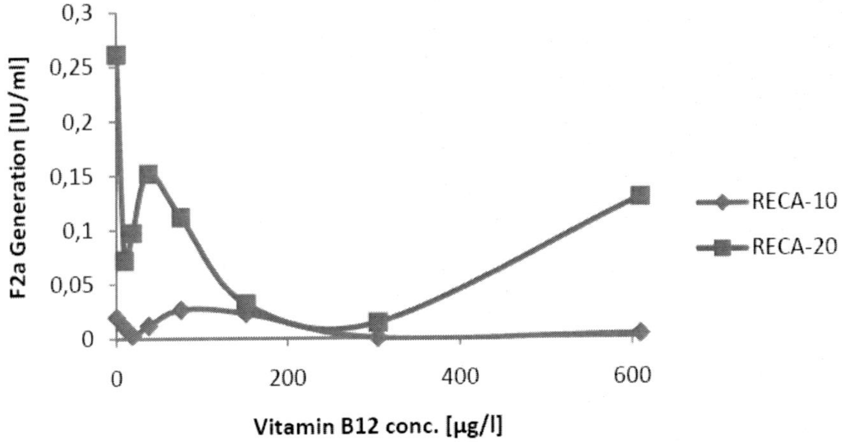

Figure 12. IC50 determination in plasma 11.

40 µl citrated plasma 11, supplemented with 0-610 µg/l cyanocobalamin, were recalcified and the thrombin generation was stopped after 10 min or 20 min by arginine as described under Methods. The approx. IC50 was 5 µg/l.

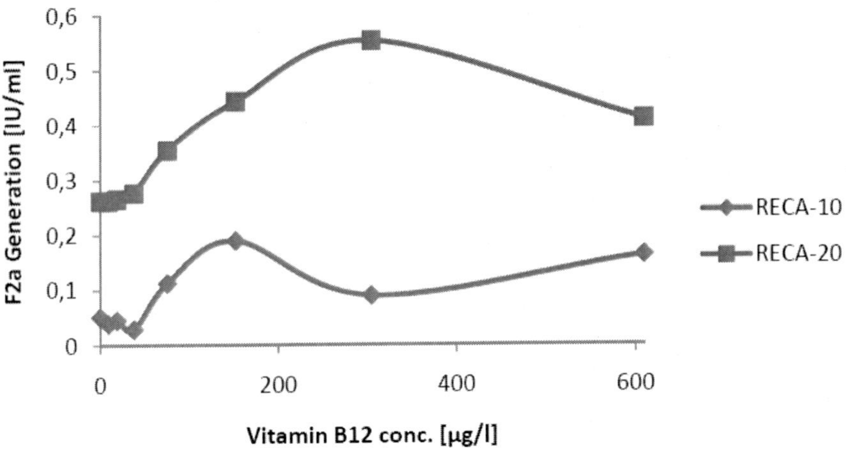

Figure 13. SC200 determination in plasma 12.

40 µl citrated plasma 12, supplemented with 0-610 µg/l cyanocobalamin, were recalcified and the thrombin generation was stopped after 10 min or 20 min by arginine as described under Methods. The approx. SC200 was 65 µg/l.

References

[1] www.wikipedia.org

[2] O Proinsias K, Giedyk M, Gryko D. Vitamin B_{12}: chemical modifications. *Chem Soc Rev*. 2013; 42: 6605-19.

[3] Jayaram N, Rao MG, Narasimha A, Raveendranathan D, Varambally S, Venkatasubramanian G, Gangadhar BN. Vitamin B_{12} levels and psychiatric symptomatology: a case series. *J Neuropsychiatry Clin Neurosci*. 2013; 25: 150-2.

[4] Glier MB, Green TJ, Devlin AM. Methyl nutrients, DNA methylation, and cardiovascular disease. *Mol Nutr Food Res*. 2014; 58: 172-82.

[5] www.AOK.de

[6] Stief TW. Drug - induced thrombin generation : the breakthrough. *Hemostasis Laboratory* 2010; 3: 3-6.

[7] Stief TW. Xenobiotic - induced pancreas carcinoma following mesenteric vein thrombosis : a hypothesis. *Hemostasis Laboratory* 2010; 3: 253-8.

[8] Stief TW. Factor 12 activation in two purified systems. *Hemostasis Laboratory* 2011; 4: 385-408.

[9] Stief TW. Zn^{2+}, hexane, or glucose activate factor 12 and/or prekallikrein in two purified systems. *Hemostasis Laboratory* 2011; 4: 409-26.

[10] Stief TW. Zn^{2+}, hexane, valproate, or glucose in two purified systems of F12-PK-HMWK. *Hemostasis Laboratory* 2012; 5: 35-50.

[11] Stief TW, Mohrez M. HMWK increases of decreases F12a generation dependent on the contact trigger concentration in two purified systems. *Hemostasis Laboratory* 2012; 5: 51-65.

[12] Stief TW. Pathological thrombin generation by the synthetic inhibitor argatroban. *Hemostasis Laboratory* 2009; 2: 83-104

[13] Stief TW, Brödje D. Thrombin generation by 3-hydroxy-butyrate, acetoacetate, or acetone. *Hemostasis Laboratory* 2013; 6: 17-50.

[14] Stief TW. Thrombin generation by creatinine. *Hemostasis Laboratory* 2011; 4: 191-9.

[15] Stief TW. Thrombin generation by therapeutic fibrinogen. *Hemostasis Laboratory* 2011; 4: 467-82.

[16] Stief TW. LMWH - action-monitoring for all patients. *Acta Paediatr*. 2012; 101: e314. 10.1111/j.1651-2227.2012.02712.x.

In: Clotting Disorders
Editor: Jeffrey L. Wilson

ISBN: 978-1-63482-830-7

Chapter 5

Using Thrombelastography or Thromboelastometry to Detect Hypercoagulable States and Predict Risks for Thromboembolic Complications

Jianyi Yin, Yousheng Li and Jieshou Li
Department of Surgery, Jinling Hospital, Nanjing University School of Medicine, Nanjing, China

Abstract

Thromboembolic complications such as deep vein thrombosis (DVT), pulmonary embolism (PE), myocardial infarction (MI) and ischemic stroke are associated with considerable morbidity and mortality. Hypercoagulability can be a great contributor to the development of thromboembolic events. Unfortunately, commonly used conventional coagulation tests such as prothrombin time (PT), international normalized ratio (INR), activated partial thromboplastin time (aPTT), platelet count and fibrinogen level are insensitive in detecting hypercoagulable states, and therefore have limited value in identifying patients with increased risks for thromboembolic complications.

Thrombelastography (TEG) and rotational thromboelastometry (ROTEM) are viscoelastic hemostatic assays that allow point-of-care description of the entire hemostatic process from clot formation to fibrinolysis. In recent years, there has been increasing evidence in the literature showing that TEG and ROTEM are reliable tools to evaluate hypercoagulable states in a variety of patient populations. Additionally, several studies have demonstrated the association of abnormal TEG or ROTEM findings and increased incidence of thromboembolic events, suggesting the predictive value of TEG and ROTEM for thromboembolic complications.

This chapter starts with a description of the methodology of viscoelastic hemostatic assay, followed by a review of literature on the utilization of TEG or ROTEM in assessing hypercoagulable states and predicting thromboembolic complications in a diverse population of medical, surgical, and trauma patients. Finally, the role of TEG and ROTEM to monitor or guide prophylaxis/treatment of thromboembolic events and the limitations of using them to detect hypercoagulability and identify patients with increased risks for thromboembolic complications are discussed.

Viscoelastic Hemostatic Assay: Overview

Viscoelastic hemostatic assay (VHA) is a point-of-care (POC) test that presents a comprehensive analysis of the entire hemostatic process from clot formation to fibrinolysis. There are two commercially available VHA systems: thrombelastography (TEG) and rotational thromboelastometry (ROTEM). Both TEG and ROTEM assess the viscoelastic properties of a blood clot based on the technique described by Hartert in 1948 [1]. VHA tests have been used to monitor coagulation function for longer than 60 years [2], but it is the recent technical innovations that have significantly improved the utilization of them in a variety of clinical scenarios.

In both TEG and ROTEM systems, whole blood sample was added into a cylindrical cup. A pin connected to a mechanical-electrical transducer via a torsion wire is suspended in the cup. As the cup (TEG) or the pin (ROTEM) oscillates in a set arc, the torque of the pin is altered due to increased strength of blood clot. This change is converted into electrical signals, which are analyzed by a computer to produce graphical and numerical results.

Despite the differences in operating characteristics and nomenclature, TEG and ROTEM are actually providing the same information with regard to the speed of coagulation initiation, clot formation kinetics, clot strength, and clot dissolution. Each part of TEG and ROTEM graph represents a specific stage of the hemostatic process, as well as each TEG and ROTEM parameter.

A representative tracing graph of TEG is shown in Figure 1. The definition and indication of TEG and ROTEM parameters is summarized in Table 1.

In recent years, VHA tests have been increasingly used for evaluation of hemostatic function in a variety of patient populations, demonstrating several advantages over conventional coagulation tests such as prothrombin time (PT), international normalized ratio (INR), activated partial thromboplastin time (aPTT), platelet count and fibrinogen level [3]. Of note, there is increasing evidence in the literature suggesting VHA tests as useful tools to detect hypercoagulable states in diverse patient populations. Moreover, several studies have demonstrated the potential of VHA tests to identify patients with increased risks for thromboembolic complications. The use of TEG and ROTEM to evaluate hypercoagulable states and predict thromboembolic complications in medical, surgical, and trauma patients is discussed below.

Use of VHA Tests to Detect Hypercoagulable States and Predict Risks for Thromboembolic Complications

Use of VHA Tests in Medical Patients

Ischemic events occur after percutaneous coronary intervention (PCI) despite standard anti-platelet treatment [4]. It has been reported that approximately 8-20% of patients receiving dual antiplatelet therapy (aspirin plus clopidogrel) had recurrent ischemic or thrombotic complications after PCI [5-7]. The role of TEG to predict post-stenting ischemic events was investigated by a series of studies from Gurbel and colleagues. In 2005, the group reported that great clot strength and rapid fibrin formation evidenced by TEG were risk factors for post-stenting ischemic events [8]. In this 6-month study including 192 post-PCI patients, of which all were on aspirin and 84% were on clopidogrel, the 38 patients developing ischemic events after PCI were found to have significantly higher MA (74 mm vs. 65 mm, $p<0.001$) and shorter R (4.3 min vs. 5.9 min, $p<0.001$) than those without post-stenting ischemic events. In another long-term follow-up study [9], the prognostic value for post-stenting ischemic events of adenosine diphosphate (ADP)-induced MA (MA_{ADP}) and thrombin-induced MA ($MA_{THROMBIN}$) was assessed over 3 years in 225 patients treated with dual-antiplatelet therapy consisting of aspirin and clopidogrel. The results revealed that patients with post-stenting ischemic events had significantly higher MA_{ADP} and $MA_{THROMBIN}$ compared to those without ischemic events ($p<0.0001$). MA_{ADP} >47 mm had the best prognostic value for long-term ischemic events, with an area under the curve of 0.84. Furthermore, MA_{ADP}>47 mm and $MA_{THROMBIN}$>69 mm were significant independent predictors of first ischemic events during the study period. These findings indicated the potential of TEG to predict ischemic events in post-stenting patients.

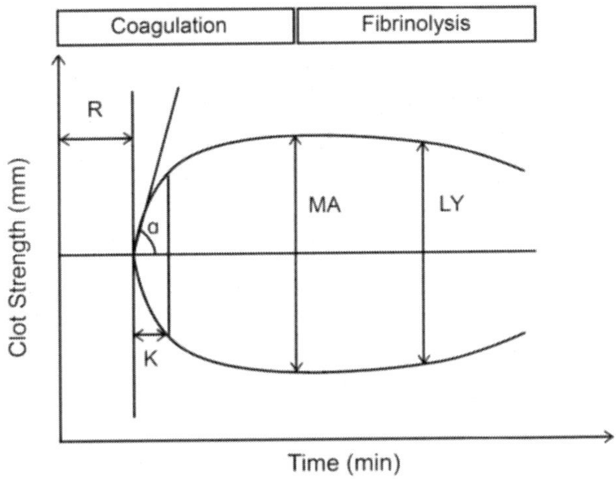

Figure 1. A representative tracing graph of TEG. R: reaction time; K: kinetics; α: α angle; MA: maximum amplitude; LY: clot lysis.

Table 1. TEG and ROTEM parameters: definition and indication

TEG	ROTEM	Definition	Underlying hemostatic process
R	CT	Time to reach an amplitude of 2 mm	Activation of enzymatic clotting factors and initial fibrin formation
K	CFT	Time to increase the amplitude from 2 mm to 20 mm	Clot formation
α	α	Slope between R and K	Clot formation
MA	MCF	Maximum amplitude of the clot	Fibrin and platelet bonding
LY	LI	% reduction in the amplitude at a specific time point	Fibrinolysis

The predictive value of TEG for ischemic events was also determined in patients with ischemic stroke by a number of studies. The first study investigating the association of TEG finding and cerebrovascular ischemic disease was reported in 1974, showing that approximately one third of patients with cerebral infarction were hypercoagulable as detected by TEG compared to normal controls within 24-48 hours after onset of stroke [10]. This finding was corroborated by a recent study enrolling 56 patients with acute ischemic stroke, which revealed that these patients had significantly shorter R (4.8 min vs. 6.0 min), greater α angle (65.0 vs. 61.5), and shorter K (1.7 min vs. 2.1 min) at admission compared to normal controls [11]. In addition, treatment with tissue plasminogen activator (t-PA) resulted in significant reduction of G (9.97 dyn/cm^2 vs. 1.29 dyn/cm^2), a computer-generated parameter reflecting the complete strength of blood clot, as well as MA (65.21 mm vs. 15.62 mm) and LY30 (0% vs. 94.4%), indicating the usefulness of TEG to monitor t-PA therapy. In a more recent prospective study including 211 patients with acute ischemic stroke, Yao et al. [12] analyzed the coagulation profile on anti-platelet treatment using TEG, and found a trend towards higher incidence of ischemic events (including ischemic stroke, myocardial infarction, and vascular death) within 1 year after stroke in patients in the higher tertile of MA. Elevated MA level was also found to be an independent predictor for poor functional outcome as defined by modified Rankin Scale≥2 (OR=1.192, p=0.022).

Use of VHA Tests in Surgical Patients

Major surgery may result in a post-operative hypercoagulable state by activating platelet, reducing anti-coagulants, compromising fibrinolysis, and activating inflammation [13]. A hypercoagulable state is associated with increased risks for thromboembolic complications, which further contribute greatly to post-operative morbidity and mortality [14]. However, reducing post-operative thromboembolic complications is challenging. Considerable variability exists in the incidence of post-operative thromboembolic events between different surgical patient populations [15], but screening tools are lacking in identifying high-risk patients. In addition, although routine thromboembolic prophylaxis is recommended for high-risk patients, post-operative thromboembolic events may still occur due to individual variability in responsiveness to prophylactic regimens.

It has been shown that the hemostatic change towards a hypercoagulable state may not be accurately described by conventional coagulation tests. As such, several studies compared VHA tests to conventional coagulation tests in evaluating coagulation profile in patients undergoing major surgeries and demonstrated VHA test as better indicator of post-operative hypercoagulable state. For example, De Pietri et al., [16] used TEG and conventional coagulation tests to assess hemostatic function in a group of patients undergoing liver (n=38) and pancreas (n=18) oncology surgeries on the day of operation and post-operative day 1, 3, 5, and 10. While conventional coagulation tests showing hypocoagulability in the post-operative period, as suggested by increased PT and INR, reduced antithrombin III level and platelet count, and normal aPTT and fibrinogen level, TEG detected a transient hypercoagulable state on post-operative day 1, as evidenced by shortened R. This study demonstrated that TEG might be superior to conventional coagulation tests as a tool to detect post-operative hypercoagulable states in surgical patients.

The ability of TEG or ROTEM to identify patients at high risks for post-operative thromboembolic events was investigated by several studies. In a prospective study of 200 consecutive patients undergoing coronary artery bypass grafting (CABG) surgery, 87 (43.5%) patients were found to be hypercoagulable by TEG before surgery (defined as MA≥69 mm). These hypercoagulable patients had higher rate of MI (6.9% vs. 3.7%), stroke (8.0% vs. 2.8%), and mortality (4.6% vs. 0.9%) than those normocoagulable patients within 30 days after surgery. The 30-day combined event rate of MI, stroke and mortality was significantly higher in hypercoagulable patients than normocoagulable patients (17.2% vs. 6.6%), and TEG-evidenced hypercoagulability was significantly associated with 30-day combined event rate in univariate analysis [17]. Similarly, in a prospective study including 313 patients undergoing major non-cardiac surgery, Hincker et al., [18] performed preoperative analysis of extrinsic rotational thromboelastometry (EXTEM), intrinsic rotational thromboelastometry (INTEM), and fibrinogen rotational thromboelastometry (FIBTEM). The study found that the 10 patients developing post-operative thromboembolic complications (including arterial or deep venous thrombosis, catheter thrombosis, and pulmonary embolism) had significantly shorter clot formation time and greater α angle and maximum clot firmness compared to those without thromboembolic complications, suggesting the value of ROTEM assay in predicting post-operative thromboembolic complications. Furthermore, McCrath and colleagues [19] performed TEG immediately after surgery in 240 surgical patients, and found that the combined incidence of post-operative thromboembolic complications including DVT, PE, ischemic stroke and MI was significantly higher in patients with MA>68 mm than those with MA≤68 mm (8.4% vs. 1.4%, p=0.016), and elevated MA was an independent predictor of post-operative MI (p=0.013). Despite the variability in study population and study design, these studies showed that VHA tests might serve as screening tools to identify patients at increased risks for post-operative thromboembolic events.

A systematic review by Dai et al. [15] provided a comprehensive evaluation of the prognostic role of TEG for post-operative thromboembolic events. The systematic review included a total of 10 studies, of which the majority confirmed the predictive value of TEG. An analysis of 5 studies reporting the diagnostic accuracy of TEG test revealed sensitivity ranging from 0% to 100% and specificity ranging from 62% to 92%. The diagnostic odds ratio ranged from 1.5 to 27.7, with an area under the curve ranging from 0.57 to 0.91. MA was found to be the best indicator of hypercoagulable states and thromboembolic events. However, these results must be interpreted with caution given the considerable variability in quality and design between the included studies. Nevertheless, this systematic review provides a specific direction for future studies to confirm the value of TEG to detect post-operative hypercoagulable states and predict risks for thromboembolic events in surgical patients.

Use of VHA Tests in Trauma Patients

In recent years, VHA tests have been increasingly used in trauma care, in particular for diagnosing and treating patients with acute trauma coagulopathy. Furthermore, there has been increasing evidence showing the potential of VHA tests to guide blood transfusion during initial resuscitation in trauma patients. Several studies have demonstrated the potential of blood transfusion protocols based on VHA tests to reduce the consumption of component blood products in trauma management [20, 21].

Apart from acute trauma coagulopathy, trauma patients may also suffer from hypercoagulability. Potentially as a physiologic response to injury and blood loss, a hypercoagulable state may be associated with increased risks for thromboembolic events. As a matter of fact, major trauma is reported to increase the risk for venous thromboembolism by 10-fold [22], and the incidence of symptomatic venous thromboembolisms can be as high as 7% regardless of medical or mechanical prophylaxis [23].

A number of studies investigated the use of VHA tests for detection of hypercoagulable states in trauma patients. For instance, Kaufmann et al. [24] used TEG for initial evaluation of coagulation function in 69 adult blunt trauma patients and found 45 of them hypercoagulable (defined as having at least two of the following TEG findings: shortened R and/or K, increased α angle, and increased MA). In another prospective cohort study including 65 trauma patients, TEG identified 62% and 26% of patients to be hypercoagulable (defined as R<3.7 min) on post-injury day 1 and day 4, respectively. However, platelet count, INR, and aPTT were within normal range during the study period, suggesting TEG as a better test for evaluation of hypercoagulability in this setting [25]. In addition, Park et al. [26] investigated the hemostatic profile of trauma patients (non-burn trauma patients, n=33, burn patients, n=25) and healthy controls (n=20) using TEG and conventional coagulation tests. While TEG suggested hypercoagulability in trauma patients, as evidenced by greater α angle and MA compared to healthy controls, PT and aPTT were prolonged in these trauma patients, indicating hypocoagulability. This finding suggested the failure of conventional coagulation tests to detect hypercoagulability and the superiority of TEG for evaluation of hypercoagulability in trauma management.

However, can VHA tests identify trauma patients at increased risks for thromboembolic complications? In a study enrolling 2070 consecutive trauma patients from a major trauma center, Cotton et al. [27] tested whether rapid TEG could predict the occurrence of PE during patients' hospital stay. The results revealed that patients developing PE (n=53) had significantly higher MA at admission (66 mm vs. 63 mm, p=0.05) compared those who did not (n=2017). After controlling for risk factors such as gender, race, age and ISS, elevated admission MA level was found to be an independent indicator of PE, with an odds ratio of 3.5 for MA>65 mm and 5.8 for MA>72 mm. In another cohort study including 152 critically ill patients, 16 of 86 patients (19%) with a hypercoagulable state (defined as G>12.4 dyn/cm^2 by rapid TEG) had thromboembolic events such as DVT and PE, whereas no patients with a normocoagulable state had any thromboembolic event (p<0.001) [28]. Elevated G value was shown to be the greatest predictor of thromboembolic events after adjustment for the presence of prophylaxis (odds ratio: 1.25, 95% confidence interval: 1.12-1.39). There was a 25% increase in odds of thromboembolic events with every 1 dyn/cm^2 increase in G value. These studies demonstrate the usefulness of TEG to predict thromboembolic complications in trauma patients.

Use of VHA Tests to Monitor or Guide Prophylaxis/Treatment of Thromboembolic Events

It has been known that individual variability exists in responsiveness to anti-thromboembolic prophylactic or therapeutic regimens. This may explain the occurrence of thromboembolic events in a subgroup of patients despite the administration of standard anti-thromboembolic prophylaxis or treatment [29]. As such, a standard dosing may not be suitable for all patients, and personalized anti-thromboembolic prophylaxis or treatment based on the evaluation of on-treatment hemostatic function may have the potential to decrease thromboembolic events and improve clinical outcomes.

The question whether VHA tests are able to monitor or guide prophylaxis or treatment of thromboembolic events were investigated by a number of studies. For example, White et al. [30] found positive correlation between dose per kg of enoxaparin and R value of TEG (p=0.011) in a series of patients admitted to coronary care unit on therapeutic use of enoxaparin (1 mg/kg twice daily), suggesting the value of TEG in monitoring low molecular weight heparin therapy. In a case study, Lombard et al. [31] described two patients who underwent stent-assisted cerebral aneurysm coil embolization and developed ischemic stroke after the procedure. Both patients received abciximab rescue treatment (initial bolus of 0.25 mg/kg followed by 12-hour infusion of 0.125 mcg/kg/minute), and TEG detected elevated MA prior to abciximab treatment in both of them. However, one patient showed decreased MA followed by complete clinical recovery rapidly after treatment, whereas the other patient had consistently elevated MA and poor neurological outcome. This study demonstrated the variability among patients in responsiveness to abciximab and indicated the potential of TEG to personalize dosing. In another case report, Ploppa et al. [32] described a patient with massive pulmonary embolism and cardiac arrest after Whipple surgery. The patient was first given 50 mg recombinant tissue plasminogen activator (rt-PA), which was the recommended maximal dose. However, TEG detected no fibrinolysis, indicating failure of thrombolytic therapy. Therefore, the patient was given another bolus of 25 mg rt-PA, after which TEG showed signs of fibrinolysis. This case study indicated that the recommended dosing of thrombolytic treatment might not be suitable in all patients, and TEG might be useful to guide dose adjustment in case of failure of standard dosing regimens.

Apart from the above reports, however, studies evaluating the use of TEG or ROTEM to guide prophylaxis or therapy of thromboembolic events are scarce in the literature [33]. Further investigations are needed to determine whether anti-thromboembolic prophylactic/therapeutic protocols based on VHA tests can reduce the incidence of thromboembolic events and improve clinical outcomes.

Limitations

Several limitations need to be considered of using TEG or ROTEM as a tool to detect hypercoagulability and identify patients at high risks for thromboembolic events. The first limitation comes from the technical nature of VHA tests. In specific, VHA systems require daily calibration, and tests should be performed by trained personnel to ensure quality of results. Moreover, technical variations (eg. use of anticoagulant and activator) must be considered when interpreting the results [34].

Second, while there is increasing evidence showing the potential of TEG or ROTEM to detect hypercoagulable states and predict thromboembolic complications, it is noteworthy that many of these studies are limited by their retrospective nature and small sample size. More importantly, considerable variability exists among these studies, making it challenging to interpret the results [15]. Further studies of high quality are needed to confirm the findings.

Third, details remain to be determined to use TEG or ROTEM as a screening tool to identify patients with high risks for thromboembolic events. For example, the parameter that has the best predictive value, the best timing of test (eg. pre- or post-operation), and the use of activator have to be decided. Furthermore, the cutoff value should be determined by further studies in different patient populations and clinical settings.

Conclusion

In sum, there has been increasing evidence in the literature showing that TEG and ROTEM may serve as reliable tools to detect hypercoagulable states in a diverse group of medical, surgical, and trauma patients. Abnormal TEG or ROTEM findings may be associated with higher risks for thromboembolic events, making them useful screening methods to identify patients with increased risks for thromboembolic complications. However, further studies of good quality are needed to confirm these findings, and studies are merited to demonstrate whether personalized anti-thromboembolic prophylactic/ therapeutic protocols based on VHA tests are safe and effective in reducing the incidence of thromboembolic complications and improving clinical outcomes.

References

[1] Hartert, H. Blood coagulation studies using thromboelastography, a new evaluation technique (in German). *Klin Wochenschr.*, 1948, 26, 577-83.

[2] De Nicola, P; Mazzetti, GM. Evaluation of thrombelastography. *Am J Clin Pathol.*, 1955, 23(4), 447-52.

[3] Yeung, MC; Tong, SY; Tong, PY; Cheung, BH; Ng, JY; Leung, GK. Use of viscoelastic haemostatic assay in emergency and elective surgery. *Hong Kong Med J.*, 2015, 21(1), 45-51.

[4] Steinhubl, SR; Berger, PB; Mann, JT; 3rd. Fry, ET; DeLago, A; Wilmer, C; et al. Early and sustained dual oral antiplatelet therapy following percutaneous coronary intervention: a randomized controlled trial. *JAMA.*, 2002, 288(19), 2411-20.

[5] Gurbel, PA; Bliden, KP; Hayes, KM; Yoho, JA; Herzog, WR; Tantry, US. The relation of dosing to clopidogrel responsiveness and the incidence of high post-treatment platelet aggregation in patients undergoing coronary stenting. *J Am Coll Cardiol.*, 2005, 45(9), 1392-6.

[6] Gurbel, PA; Bliden, KP; Hiatt, BL; O'Connor, CM. Clopidogrel for coronary stenting: response variability, drug resistance, and the effect of pretreatment platelet reactivity. *Circulation.*, 2003, 107(23), 2908-13.

[7] Mehta, SR; Yusuf, S; Peters, RJ; Bertrand, ME; Lewis, BS; Natarajan, MK; et al. Effects of pretreatment with clopidogrel and aspirin followed by long-term therapy in patients undergoing percutaneous coronary intervention: the PCI-CURE study. *Lancet.*, 2001, 358(9281), 527-33.

[8] Gurbel, PA; Bliden, KP; Guyer, K; Cho, PW; Zaman, KA; Kreutz, RP; et al. Platelet reactivity in patients and recurrent events post-stenting: results of the PREPARE POST-STENTING Study. *J Am Coll Cardiol.*, 2005, 46(10), 1820-6.

[9] Gurbel, PA; Bliden, KP; Navickas, IA; Mahla, E; Dichiara, J; Suarez, TA; et al. Adenosine diphosphate-induced platelet-fibrin clot strength: a new thrombelastographic indicator of long-term poststenting ischemic events. *Am Heart J.*, 2010, 160(2), 346-54.

[10] Ettinger, M. Thromboelastographic studies in cerebral infarction. *Stroke*., 1974, 5(3), 350-4.

[11] Elliott, A; Wetzel, J; Roper, T; Pivalizza, E; McCarthy, J; Wallace, C; et al. Thromboelastography in patients with acute ischemic stroke. *Int J Stroke*., 2015, 10(2), 194-201.

[12] Yao, X; Dong, Q; Song, Y; Wang, Y; Deng, Y; Li, Y. Thrombelastography maximal clot strength could predict one-year functional outcome in patients with ischemic stroke. *Cerebrovasc Dis*., 2014, 38(3), 182-90.

[13] Gibbs, NM; Crawford, GP; Michalopoulos, N. Postoperative changes in coagulant and anticoagulant factors following abdominal aortic surgery. *J Cardiothorac Vasc Anesth*., 1992, 6(6), 680-5.

[14] Nerurkar, J; Wade, WE; Martin, BC. Cost/death averted with venous thromboembolism prophylaxis in patients undergoing total knee replacement or knee arthroplasty. *Pharmacotherapy*., 2002, 22(8), 990-1000.

[15] Dai, Y; Lee, A; Critchley, LA; White, PF. Does thromboelastography predict postoperative thromboembolic events? A systematic review of the literature. *Anesth Analg*., 2009, 108(3), 734-42.

[16] De, Pietri, L; Montalti, R; Begliomini, B; Scaglioni, G; Marconi, G; Reggiani, A; et al. Thromboelastographic changes in liver and pancreatic cancer surgery: hypercoagulability, hypocoagulability or normocoagulability? *Eur J Anaesthesiol*., 2010, 27(7), 608-16.

[17] Rafiq, S; Johansson, PI; Ostrowski, SR; Stissing, T; Steinbruchel, DA. Hypercoagulability in patients undergoing coronary artery bypass grafting: prevalence, patient characteristics and postoperative outcome. *Eur J Cardiothorac Surg*., 2012, 41(3), 550-5.

[18] Hincker, A; Feit, J; Sladen, RN; Wagener, G. Rotational thromboelastometry predicts thromboembolic complications after major non-cardiac surgery. *Crit Care*., 2014, 18(5), 549.

[19] McCrath, DJ; Cerboni, E; Frumento, RJ; Hirsh, AL; Bennett-Guerrero, E. Thromboelastography maximum amplitude predicts postoperative thrombotic complications including myocardial infarction. *Anesth Analg*., 2005, 100(6), 1576-83.

[20] Yin, J; Zhao, Z; Li, Y; Wang, J; Yao, D; Zhang, S; et al. Goal-directed transfusion protocol via thrombelastography in patients with abdominal trauma: a retrospective study. *World J Emerg Surg*., 2014, 9:28.

[21] Kashuk, JL; Moore, EE; Wohlauer, M; Johnson, JL; Pezold, M; Lawrence, J; et al. Initial experiences with point-of-care rapid

thrombelastography for management of life-threatening postinjury coagulopathy. *Transfusion.*, 2012, 52(1), 23-33.
[22] McLaughlin, DF; Wade, CE; Champion, HR; Salinas, J; Holcomb, JB. Thromboembolic complications following trauma. *Transfusion.*, 2009, 49 Suppl 5, 256S-63S.
[23] Shackford, SR; Davis, JW; Hollingsworth-Fridlund, P; Brewer, NS; Hoyt, DB; Mackersie, RC. Venous thromboembolism in patients with major trauma. *Am J Surg.*, 1990, 159(4), 365-9.
[24] Kaufmann, CR; Dwyer, KM; Crews, JD; Dols, SJ; Trask, AL. Usefulness of thrombelastography in assessment of trauma patient coagulation. *J Trauma.*, 1997, 42(4), 716-20, discussion 20-2.
[25] Schreiber, MA; Differding, J; Thorborg, P; Mayberry, JC; Mullins, RJ. Hypercoagulability Is Most Prevalent Early after Injury and in Female Patients. *J Trauma.*, 2005, 58(3), 475-81.
[26] Park, MS; Martini, WZ; Dubick, MA; Salinas, J; Butenas, S; Kheirabadi, BS; et al. Thromboelastography as a better indicator of hypercoagulable state after injury than prothrombin time or activated partial thromboplastin time. *J Trauma.*, 2009, 67(2), 266-75, discussion 75-6.
[27] Cotton, BA; Minei, KM; Radwan, ZA; Matijevic, N; Pivalizza, E; Podbielski, J; et al. Admission rapid thrombelastography predicts development of pulmonary embolism in trauma patients. *J Trauma Acute Care Surg.*, 2012, 72(6), 1470-5, discussion 5-7.
[28] Kashuk, JL; Moore, EE; Sabel, A; Barnett, C; Haenel, J; Le, T; et al. Rapid thrombelastography (r-TEG) identifies hypercoagulability and predicts thromboembolic events in surgical patients. *Surgery.*, 2009, 146(4), 764-72, discussion 72-4.
[29] Malinoski, D; Jafari, F; Ewing, T; Ardary, C; Conniff, H; Baje, M; et al. Standard prophylactic enoxaparin dosing leads to inadequate anti-Xa levels and increased deep venous thrombosis rates in critically ill trauma and surgical patients. *J Trauma.*, 2010, 68(4), 874-80.
[30] White, H; Sosnowski, K; Bird, R; Jones, M; Solano, C. The utility of thromboelastography in monitoring low molecular weight heparin therapy in the coronary care unit. *Blood Coagul Fibrinolysis.*, 2012, 23(4), 304-10.
[31] Lombard, FW; Welsby, IJ; Alexander, MJ; Borel, CO. Thromboelastography detects inadequate response to abciximab therapy during stent-assisted cerebral aneurysm coil embolization complicated by stroke. *Neurocrit Care.*, 2006, 4(1), 32-4.

[32] Ploppa, A; Unertl, KE; Nohe, B. Thrombelastometry-guided thrombolytic therapy in massive pulmonary artery embolism. *Acta Anaesthesiol Scand.*, 2010, 54(9), 1145-8.

[33] Rafiq, S; Johansson, PI; Zacho, M; Stissing, T; Kofoed, K; Lilleor, NB; et al. Thrombelastographic haemostatic status and antiplatelet therapy after coronary artery bypass surgery (TEG-CABG trial): assessing and monitoring the antithrombotic effect of clopidogrel and aspirin versus aspirin alone in hypercoagulable patients: study protocol for a randomized controlled trial. *Trials.*, 2012, 13, 48.

[34] da Luz, LT; Nascimento, B, Fau - Rizoli, S; Rizoli, S. Thrombelastography (TEG(R)): practical considerations on its clinical use in trauma resuscitation. *Scand J Trauma Resusc Emerg Med.*, 2013, 21, 29.

In: Clotting Disorders
Editor: Jeffrey L. Wilson

ISBN: 978-1-63482-830-7

Chapter 6

Prophylactic Fresh Frozen Plasma: Time for a Re-Think?

Anita Sugavanam[1] **and Susan V. Mallett**[2]*

[1]Anaesthetic Consultant, Brighton and Sussex University Hospitals, Brighton, East Sussex, UK

[2]Anaesthetic Consultant, Royal Free Hospital NHS Foundation Trust, Pond St, London, UK

Abstract

Practice guidelines continue to give somewhat conflicting advice regarding indications for Fresh Frozen Plasma (FFP) transfusion and it is therefore not surprising that repeatedly worldwide, audits of FFP usage demonstrate abundant inappropriate transfusion. Nearly half of all FFP transfusions are given prophylactically in order to correct prolonged prothrombin time (PT) and/or international normalized ratio (INR) prior to an invasive or operative procedure in the absence of bleeding. However, the evidence supporting this practice is very poor and will be reviewed in this chapter. Meta-analyses fail to demonstrate that elevated PT and/or INR predict(s) bleeding across a wide range of specialties. Global assays of hemostasis such as viscoelastography may be more useful in predicting bleeding risk but large-scale outcome studies are required. Studies in different patient populations show that coagulation

* Correspondance to Anita Sugavanam: anita.sugavanam@nhs.net

factor levels are generally well above the threshold for adequate hemostasis (30%) until the INR exceeds 2.0 x control. In addition, FFP does not reliably correct INR values ≤ 1.8 x control unless given in volumes much larger than conventional doses. Specific clinical scenarios where prophylactic FFP transfusions often occur include patients with liver disease, procedures in critical care, cardiac and liver surgery and warfarin reversal. There is little evidence to support plasma transfusion in any of these situations and the risks of transfusion are not insignificant, including transfusion related acute lung injury (TRALI), transfusion associated circulatory overload (TACO), delays in procedures and increased cost. Clinical trials looking at bleeding risks with or without plasma transfusion have been difficult to carry out and the challenges encountered will be reviewed in this chapter. Deeply-engrained personal beliefs and lack of evidence continue to fuel prophylactic FFP transfusion by clinicians; the call for clinical trials has never been greater.

1. Introduction

It is now a requirement of good clinical practice to minimize the unnecessary and inappropriate use of blood and blood products. Patient blood management programs are now addressing this issue, but the focus remains primarily on red blood cell usage. The worldwide use of fresh frozen plasma (FFP), particularly for prophylactic and pre-procedural reasons, remains inordinately high, and has not decreased over the last ten years to any significant extent, in contrast to the falling use of red blood cells as restrictive transfusion thresholds are increasingly adopted (1). A recent retrospective study showed an unchanging rate of FFP use in over 40 hospitals in the US over an eight year period, even though FFP is no longer recommended in many clinical scenarios(2).

A significant proportion of FFP is given prophylactically on the assumption that prolonged coagulation tests, such as prothrombin time (PT), activated partial thromboplastin time (aPTT) and international normalized ratio (INR) predict an increased bleeding risk, and that FFP transfusion will correct these tests and consequently reduce bleeding risk. This review, which focuses only on the use of FFP in patients who are not actively bleeding, critically questions these assumptions in the context of pre-procedural administration of FFP, and also examines why carrying out high quality trials in this area has been so problematic.

2. Current Practice in FFP Transfusion

Worldwide, FFP is given for two primary indications; prevention of bleeding (prophylactic) or treatment of bleeding (therapeutic). In terms of patients who are actively bleeding, guidelines are reasonably consistent, and trigger thresholds for FFP transfusion are generally set at an INR $\geq$ 1.5. Nevertheless, there is ongoing discussion as to the best trigger threshold/ target INR, and also the volume/ratio of FFP that should optimally be transfused in relation to red blood cells (3-5). There is significantly more variability in the recommendations for pre-procedural thresholds, and this is especially the case in patients with liver disease (see table 1). This is important as the prophylactic use of FFP accounts for nearly 50% of all plasma transfused (1, 6-8). There is a surprising lack of high quality evidence on which guidelines are based, and much is a reflection of expert opinion and observational studies rather than RCTs. Consequently confidence in, and compliance with, existing guidelines tends to be relatively poor (9, 10).

A panel of experts convened by the AABB reported a lack of evidence for FFP transfusion in all settings except massive transfusion and warfarin-associated intracranial hemorrhage (9). A recent systematic review of 80 randomized controlled trials (RCTs) also found a lack of evidence for both prophylactic and therapeutic FFP across a large range of clinical settings (11). The only individual RCTs in the review demonstrating beneficial effects of FFP were in plasma exchange for thrombotic thrombocytopenic purpura (TTP), treatment of early thrombocytopenia in dengue fever, and use of FFP in priming cardiac bypass pumps along with packed red cells prior to cardiac surgery in children. Of concern, in both the 2004 and updated 2012 systematic review, the authors found most trials had large methodological limitations in terms of quality assessment and reporting of adequate randomization, allocation, concealment and blinding (only two of the 21 identified trials fulfilled all criteria). In addition, most trials enrolled small numbers of patients (usually less than 30 patients), and provided inadequate information on the ability of the trial to detect meaningful differences in outcomes between the two patient groups. Doses of FFP used were variable (6-15ml/kg), and the potential for bias was usually very high. In addition, no studies took adequate account of the extent to which adverse effects might have negated the clinical benefits of treatment with FFP. A prophylactic policy aimed at preventing bleeding complications would involve transfusing a large number of patients, many of whom might not bleed even if prophylactic FFP were not given. Studies of prophylaxis must therefore also include an estimate of the adverse outcomes as well as an estimate of the proportion of patients for whom a significant bleeding problem may be prevented.

Two recent multicenter RCTs to determine if prophylactic FFP is effective in decreasing bleeding complications in patients with INR $\geq$ 1.5 were prematurely terminated due to logistics with recruitment (12-14). It appears that the practice of prophylactic transfusion in response to a prolonged PT or INR value is so engrained, and the fear of bleeding (and litigation) so great, that FFP transfusion has not yet been subjected to standard evidence-based scrutiny. Nevertheless, there is a large amount of published information available that questions the validity of these assumptions.

Despite some of the recent blood transfusion guidelines veering away from prophylactic FFP transfusion in light of a lack of evidence (9), audits repeatedly show that variable and high proportions of FFP (ranging from 26% to 83%) are given outside of current indications (6, 15-18). The most common reason for inappropriate orders is a correction of a prolonged INR in the absence of bleeding (1, 6, 15, 16). One of the largest national audits carried out looked at nearly 5000 FFP transfusions (1) and found that 43% of all adult FFP transfusions were given to patients in the absence of any documented bleeding, and that a significant proportion (27%) had a pre-transfusion INR $\leq$ 1.5. Over half of FFP transfusions given to patients on warfarin were also in the absence of bleeding. Similarly, in three prospective audits in Canada, 45% of 671 (19) 48% of 547 (20) and 28.6% of 559 (18) FFP transfusions respectively were deemed inappropriate, mainly given to non-bleeding patients with aPTT or INR values $\leq$ 1.5 x normal. Worldwide this has been a repetitive finding (21-23).. A recent multi regional audit looked specifically at blood component use in over 1300 patients with liver cirrhosis, and 76% of patients given prophylactic FFP received it prior to a procedure (24). For those undergoing a low risk procedure such as central venous catheter insertion or paracentesis, 33% had a pre-transfusion INR < 2.0.

Inappropriate transfusion amongst critically-ill patients is a more stubborn problem and a large retrospective US study of over 70000 plasma transfusions found that 80% of transfusions occurred in critical care and medical/surgical wards prior to procedures carried out in those settings rather than the operating room (8). Worldwide 20-30% of critically ill patients receive FFP during the course of their stay on intensive care (ICU) (7, 17). In this environment there is even less adherence to guidelines, wider variation in use and higher inappropriate use (7, 25, 26).

Table 1. Summary of guidelines on plasma transfusion prior to invasive procedures

	British Committee for Standards in Hematology (27)	**American Society of Anesthes-iologists (28)**	**Canadian Members of the Expert Working Group (29)**	**Australian & New Zealand Society of Blood transfusion Ltd (30)**	**French Security Agency of Health Product Safety (31)**	**German Medical Association Guidelines (32)**	**Transfusion Medicine Advisory Group (TMAG) British Columbia, Canada (33)**	**Cardiovascular and Interventional Radiological Society of Europe Endorsement (34)**
Dose	10-15mls/kg	10-15mls/kg	Not stated	10-20mls/kg	10-15mls/kg	20ml/kg	10-15ml/kg	At least 10mls/kg
In Liver Disease	May be advocated by some but response unpredictable	Not stated	If patient bleeding and PT and aPTT> trigger	May be appropriate in the presence of bleeding and abnormal coagulation	If patient bleeding and PT and aPTT> trigger	If risk of massive haemorrhage and/or coagulopathy with Quick value < 50%	Routine use questionable. Response unpredictable	Not stated
Before Invasive procedures	Not stated	Not stated	If INR > 2 for procedures such as liver biopsy, paracentesis, thoracocentes	Can be used in non-bleeding patients who are considered at risk of bleeding in association with PT/aPTT ratio >1.5 or in patients with personal or family history of bleeding	Indicated if significant risk of bleeding and coagulation triggers	Not for Liver biopsy, paracentesis, thoracocentes or central venous puncture. Not for liver transplants if Quick > 50%	Not for mild-moderately high INRs. Factor levels need to be 40%. May be more conservative in lumbar disc space injections, neurosurgery, pulmonary biopsies	"Low risk" procedures, keep INR <2 "Moderate-High Risk" procedires kep INR < 1.5

Studies of prophylaxis must therefore also include an estimate of the adverse outcomes as well as an estimate of the proportion of patients for whom a significant bleeding problem may be prevented.

Two recent multicenter RCTs to determine if prophylactic FFP is effective in decreasing bleeding complications in patients with INR ≥ 1.5 were prematurely terminated due to logistics with recruitment [12-14]. It appears that the practice of prophylactic transfusion in response to a prolonged PT or INR value is so engrained, and the fear of bleeding (and litigation) so great, that FFP transfusion has not yet been subjected to standard evidence-based scrutiny. Nevertheless, there is a large amount of published information available that questions the validity of these assumptions.

Despite some of the recent blood transfusion guidelines veering away from prophylactic FFP transfusion in light of a lack of evidence [9], audits repeatedly show that variable and high proportions of FFP (ranging from 26% to 83%) are given outside of current indications [6, 15-18]. The most common reason for inappropriate orders is a correction of a prolonged INR in the absence of bleeding [6, 15, 16] [1]. One of the largest national audits carried out looked at nearly 5000 FFP transfusions [1] and found that 43% of all adult FFFP transfusions were given to patients in the absence of any documented bleeding, and that a significant proportion (27%) had a pre-transfusion INR ≤ 1.5. Over half of FFP transfusions given to patients on warfarin were also in the absence of bleeding. Similarly, in three prospective audits in Canada, 45% of 671 [19], 48% of 547 [20] and 28.6% of 559 [18] FFP transfusions respectively were deemed inappropriate, mainly given to non-bleeding patients with aPTT or INR values ≤ 1.5 x normal. Worldwide this has been a repetitive finding. [21-23]. A recent multi regional audit looked specifically at blood component use in over 1300 patients with liver cirrhosis, and 76% of patients given prophylactic FFFP received it prior to a procedure (24). For those undergoing a low risk procedure such as central venous catheter insertion or paracentesis, 33% had a pre-transfusion INR < 2.0.

Inappropriate transfusion amongst critically-ill patients is a more stubborn problem and a large retrospective US study of over 70000 plasma transfusions found that 80% of transfusions occurred in critical care and medical/surgical wards prior to procedures carried out in those settings rather than the operating room [7]. Worldwide 20-30% of critically ill patients receive FFP during the course of their stay on intensive care (ICU) [8, 17]. In this environment there is even less adherence to guidelines, wider variation in use and higher inappropriate use [8, 21, 25, 26]. This may be because it is felt these patients are different to other hospital in-patients. Yet in the case of red cell transfusion, the principle of a restrictive policy has filtered through to clinical practice and in a recent audit of practice in 47 ICUs across Australia and New Zealand, only 2% of red cell transfusions were considered inappropriate compared to 29% of FFP transfusions (35).

ICU physicians often state bleeding as the reason for transfusion of FFP, but many of these cases are suspected or recent bleeding, or bleeding in the presence of near-normal PT-INR values. In fact physicians often do not agree on the definitions of a major bleeding episode (7) and there is little confidence in available tests to predict bleeding. It is hence unsurprising that so much FFP ends up not being given (in one survey 28% of FFP products were either returned to the transfusion center or wasted (7)). In addition, PT and/or INR values are often not re-checked within six hours after FFP transfusion (32% of cases in one national multicenter study (17)). Chronic liver disease and concurrent red cell transfusion both independently increase the likelihood of prophylactic plasma transfusion regardless of severity of prolonged PT (36).

Walsh et al. (37) looked at patients with prolonged PT values in 29 ICUs in the UK: Half (51%) of FFP transfusions were to non-bleeding patients, and there was high variability in the doses of FFP given (range 2.4 - 41.1ml/kg). PT prolongation was independently associated with higher mortality but these prolongations were often mild, short-lived and naturally corrected themselves with supportive care and treatment of the underlying condition, not with plasma transfusions. This is possibly due to correction of liver hypo-perfusion, dehydration, anemia, hypoxia, hypocalcaemia, hypothermia and acidosis. Holland and Brooks (38) also noted the corrective effect of medical treatment alone on mildly prolonged coagulation factors in stable non-bleeding hospital patients: In their observational study on the effect of FFP on INR values, 179 patients received FFP transfusions and 71 patients acted as a control group (adult patients with INR values 1.3-1.6 x control not receiving FFP transfusions). They reported that mildly elevated INRs (1.3-1.6 x control) decreased without FFP via supportive care after a median time of 8.5 hours. Another systematic review of patients with upper non-variceal gastrointestinal bleeding involving 769 patients did not find INR to predict re-bleeding but it was associated with higher mortality and was possibly more useful as a proxy of co-morbid burden (39). It must be noted alongside this, that the observed higher mortality in patients with higher PT values may partly be caused by FFP transfusions themselves.

3. Risks of FFP Transfusion

In order to be able to assess the risk benefit balance when considering whether or not to transfuse FFP, it is vital that clinicians understand the adverse effect profile of FFP. FFP and platelets are probably the blood components with the highest risk profiles (40) but hemovigilance reports vary highly and this is in part due to passive reporting systems. In France, where reporting is mandatory, the incidence of adverse reactions to FFP has been reported as 1:1700 (41) yet another analysis of over 30,000 FFP transfusions in the US reported it as high as 1:360 (42). Either way, under-reporting worldwide has maintained the practice of transfusion outside of current guidelines (43-45) as there is little appreciation of associated risk. A summary of risks is presented in Table 2.

Table 2. Associated Risks of Plasma Transfusion

- Febrile and Allergic Reaction (1-3% of FFP transfusions) (47)
- Transfusion-Associated Circulatory Overload or TACO (possibly as high as 1 in 10 transfusions in the elderly (44)
- Transfusion-related Acute Lung Injury or TRALI (estimated incidence of 6-23%) (48-50)
- Post Transfusion Purpura (51)
- Viral infection: (estimated risk of hepatitis C transmission 1:50 million and Hepatitis B 1: 1.2 million)
- Nocosomial Infections through detrimental immunomodulation (52, 53)
- Hemolytic Anaemia (ABO compatibility recommended)
-

Morbidity associated with plasma transfusion has been repetitively demonstrated, in particular multi-organ failure and acute lung injury (ALI) across a range of patients; trauma patients, massively-transfused patients, surgical, critically-ill, and pediatric patients (45). The existence and role of transfusion-related immunomodulation is still under debate, but higher pneumonia and nosocomial infection rates have been reported in transfused patients (45, 52-55). Higher rates of venous and arterial thrombosis have also been reported in children but a causal link is difficult to ascertain (2). The largest bodies of evidence regarding mortality stem from reviews of retrospective studies in massively transfused trauma patients rather than RCTs and these mostly show improved survival with aggressive plasma transfusion although the optimal FFP: RBC ratio remains unclear (56, 57). Studies in civilian trauma and non-massively transfused patients are more inconsistent, some studies showing higher, lower and unchanged mortality and teasing out confounding factors is challenging (45, 58). There is very little regarding morbidity and mortality from prophylactic FFP transfusion specifically.

Both transfusion-related acute lung injury (TRALI) and transfusion-associated circulatory overload (TACO) merit some specific consideration. TRALI (48-50) was considered the leading cause of mortality associated with blood product transfusion until recently, occurring 5-6 times more frequently with high plasma volume components such as FFP compared to red cells (59, 60). Dara et al., (61) retrospectively looked at 115 critically-ill patients where there was no difference in new bleeding episodes between those who did and did not receive FFP transfusion prior to invasive procedures, but new-onset ALI was significantly more frequent in the transfused group (18% versus 4% $p = 0.021$). The etiology of TRALI is unclear but most likely involves recipient factors which firstly prime neutrophils on pulmonary endothelium and secondly prime leukocyte antibodies in the donor plasma which then activate these neutrophils and cause a permeability edema (the so called "two hit" hypothesis)(45). There is certainly a higher degree of this allo-immunization in FFP from multiparous women (49, 62) and as a result FFP is now limited to male donors or nulliparous women in many countries. This has resulted in an impressive decline (from 1:4000 to 1:12,000 in one active surveillance study) (63) but not elimination of TRALI (60, 64).

TACO is both under-recognized and under-reported (42, 65). It has only been reported as a separate category since 2007 by the Serious Hazards Of Transfusion (SHOT) group in the UK who have seen a jump in cases per year from 40 in 2010 to 96 in 2013 [59]. The incidence in the literature varies from 1:1566 to 1:68 transfusions or 1-8% (66). This is in part due to changing definitions and recognition/reporting systems. Although often clinically difficult to distinguish from TRALI, the underlying mechanism for hypoxia is a hydrostatic edema rather than permeability one. Recipient factors such as older age, low body weight and co-existing renal/cardiac dysfunction play a role (66) but there are also transfusion factors such as volume transfused and rate of transfusion: Transfusion of as little as 500mls of fluid to patients with congestive heart failure or ischemic heart disease has been shown to increase levels of Brain Natriuretic Peptide (67) (a sensitive marker of volume overload). Of importance, TACO accounts for a large proportion of major morbidity and death associated with transfusion. In the SHOT report of 2013 16 out of 96 episodes of TACO were attributable to plasma transfusion (66) and strong recommendations were made to increase education and awareness about TACO and identify patients at risk.

4. What Is the Evidence That Prophylactic FFP Transfusion Reduces Bleeding Risk?

4a. Does a Prolonged PT and/or INR Predict an Increased Bleeding Risk in Stable Patients?

The Prothrombin Time (PT)

The conventional tests of coagulation, aPTT and PT, were developed primarily for screening patients with hereditary deficiencies of individual clotting factors or for the monitoring of anticoagulant therapy such as Vitamin K antagonists (VKA) and heparin. These tests were never intended as a model of *in vivo* hemostasis, or as screening tests for bleeding risk in the general population. PT was designed to detect deficiencies of factors II, V, VII and X and therefore to monitor anticoagulant therapy with VKAs and/or detect acquired bleeding disorders such as vitamin K deficiency (68). The aPTT was similarly designed to screen for hemophilia and other coagulation factor deficiencies (69). The endpoint of measurement in both tests is the initial formation of fibrin strands which is detected by optical or electrical means and reported in seconds (70). Neither test reflects the activity of naturally occurring anticoagulants such as antithrombin, protein C, protein S, and tissue factor pathway inhibitor (TFPI). One concern about PT is that *in vitro* it is initiated by high concentrations of tissue factor which does not reflect the lower concentrations *in vivo* (71). In addition, it is not possible to estimate overall strength and stability of the clot because these tests are terminated at very low levels of thrombin (about 5-10nM), and before fibrin is polymerized by activated factor XIII. As such they do not give any information on total thrombin generation, which relies on the balance between pro-coagulants and anti-coagulants. A prolonged aPTT, PT or INR may reflect a reduced level of pro-coagulation factors (such as in liver disease or DIC) or the presence of an inhibitor (such as acquired hemophilia, heparin, direct thrombin inhibitors and anti Xa inhibitors). This may predispose the patient to bleeding, thrombosis or no change in hemostasis despite abnormal PT/aPTT values. For example, factor XII deficiency leads to a prolonged aPTT but does not affect bleeding risk whereas factor XIII deficiency does increase bleeding risk without altering

PT or aPTT. Patients with antiphosphoplipid antibody or lupus anticoagulant may present with prolonged PT and/or aPTT values but these patients are actually at increased risk of thrombosis. It has also been repetitively shown that patients with acute and chronic liver disease who have prolonged PT or INR values may have normal or even enhanced thrombin generation (72). Finally it must not be forgotten that, pre-analytical error is the most common cause for a prolonged PT value (70): Under-filling of bottles, elevated hematocrit, anticoagulant contamination of lines and variations in instrument-reagent mixtures can all prolong the PT. It is clear there is a significant false positive and false negative rate: The false negatives render the test unhelpful and the false positive tests generate unwarranted investigations. Inappropriate FFP transfusion is associated with the possibility of adverse events, and also has a financial cost. In addition, the risk/benefit equation must involve balancing the inherent logistic issues caused by ordering, defrosting and then transfusing relatively larger volumes of FFP in stable, normovolemic patients which inevitably leads to delays in performing proposed diagnostic or therapeutic procedures, as well as putting some patients at risk of TACO.

The International Normalized ratio (INR)

The INR was developed to monitor VKA therapy and to standardize results in order to account for the highly variable sensitivities of thromboplastin reagents (human, animal or recombinant) used in different centers to measure PT. It is calculated via the formula $[\text{patient PT/mean normal PT}]^{ISI}$ where the International Sensitivity Index (ISI) is a value assigned to the thromboplastin reagent when compared with a WHO reference thromboplastin, which is assigned an ISI of 1.0. The threshold of an INR of 1.5 for an increased bleeding risk came out of studies that originally used thromboplastin reagents with high ISIs (≥ 2). Since then, manufacturers have shifted towards more sensitive (lower ISI) reagents to improve inter-laboratory INR reproducibility: Today the reagents have ISIs of 0.9-1.2 and therefore PT values are often prolonged even if factor VII levels are above 40% which is more than adequate for hemostasis (73). The PT-INR ratio literature has not taken this historical shift in thromboplastin reagent sensitivities into account. Data from studies done before the 1990's need some reconsideration. For example, McVay and colleagues observed no increased bleeding in patients with a variety of clinical conditions undergoing paracentesis and thoracocentesis if the PT ratio ≤ 2 x control ratio (74) and the same for percutaneous liver biopsy if the PT ratio ≤ 1.5 x control ratio (75). Apart from concerns about the definition of a bleed in these studies, the thromboplastin agent used at the time had an ISI index ≥ 2. This actually translates into an INR threshold range of 2.25 to 4 rather an INR of 1.5 (76) In patients with liver disease there are wide inter-laboratory variations in INR, and it has been suggested that a modified INR using plasma from patients with cirrhosis, would be more appropriate (77, 78).

The INR was calibrated to guide VKA therapy but does not reliably predict bleeding risk even in these patients as suggested by studies looking bleeding events post femoral coronary angiography (79), prostate biopsies (80) or urgent reversal prior to surgery (81). Often a critical INR value of 5 is chosen for indicating an increased risk of spontaneous bleeding but studies show there is a poor correlation with vitamin-K dependent factor levels (82) and the rate and magnitude of factor level decline with INR (83-85). Patient demographics such as age, interacting medications, presence of atrial fibrillation and co-morbidities, as well as being warfarin-naïve are all recognized predictors in patients taking VKA. Bleeding risk scores for warfarinized patients have been devised according to these criteria rather than the absolute INR value although their predictive values are still poor (86).

Clinical Trials Assessing PT-INR As Predictors of Bleeding

There is little hard evidence to support mild to moderate elevations of PT-INR as good predictors of bleeding risk (15, 68, 87). Chee et al., (88) published guidelines on the assessment of bleeding risk prior to invasive procedures in 2008 for the British Committee of Standards in Hematology (BCSH). They found only nine trials involving patients from general surgery and pediatric Ears Nose and Throat (ENT) surgery and these were mainly retrospective case series, with selection bias and imperfect recall. The calculated collective positive predictive value was poor (0.03 - 0.22) and the likelihood ratio (LR) for a positive test ranged from 0.94 to 5.10 with 95% confidence intervals crossing 1.0 in the few trials that were prospective. Segal and Dzik (87) performed a meta-analysis of 25 studies looking at coagulation tests as predictors of bleeding: In 12 out of 14 studies that included patients with normal and abnormal coagulation tests, bleeding rates are almost identical and over a range of procedures (central line placement, thoracocentesis, lumbar puncture, paracentesis, and liver biopsy) (see Figure 1). There was only one RCT, which looked at liver biopsies in 100 patients, and only 2% of patients met their bleeding endpoint criteria despite abnormal coagulation tests. The remaining studies were mainly small retrospective case series and did not report the degree of PT prolongation or have a control group. Only in one study of patients undergoing kidney biopsy were bleeding complications higher in patients with abnormal tests and in another study of transjugular liver biopsies, the number of bleeding complications was higher in patients with normal coagulation tests.

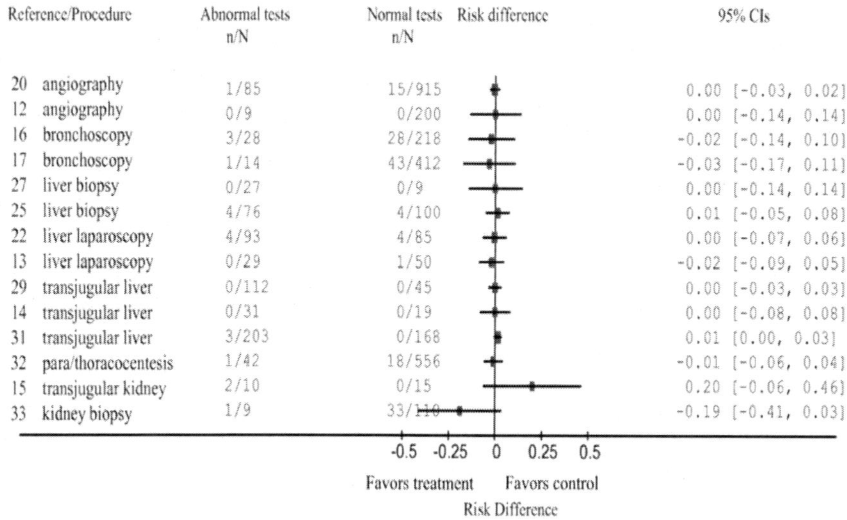

Figure 1. The absolute differences (and 95% confidence intervals) in the proportion of patients with major procedure-related bleeding in the groups with and without abnormalities of pre-procedure coagulation tests. Taken from review of 25 studies by Segal JB and Dzik WH(87).

Ng (76) reports a similar lack of evidence for PT or INR as predictors of bleeding for larger procedures such as aortic surgery, kidney transplant, head and neck surgery, craniotomy and total joint replacements. Eckman et al., (89) pooled results from observational studies in general surgery, adenotonsillectomy, angiography and gynaecological surgery and calculated that the LR for a positive coagulation test result ranged from 0 to 33 and the sensitivity of an abnormal test ranged from 0-100%. Pooling results like this does require cautious interpretation due to heterogeneity in study characteristics, definitions of bleeding outcomes and testing panels. Although the overall level of evidence is poor, these studies collectively suggest that mild to moderate elevations of PT and/or INR are not associated with a significant increase in bleeding risk. The evidence for prophylactic FFP use in specific clinical scenarios such as liver disease and procedures in critical care is outlined later in this chapter.

4b. The Relationship between PT-INR and Coagulation Factor Levels in Different Clinical Settings

Looking more closely at the relationship between coagulation factor levels and coagulation tests may help further understand the utility of these tests in assessing bleeding risk. Studies on patients with hemophilia A and B show that these patients are at increased risk of bleeding during surgery or following trauma if their factor levels fall below 30iu/dl or 30% of normal (73). With these levels of factors, they would be labeled as mild hemophiliacs who would bleed only after surgery or external trauma.

Vitamin K Deficiency

Looking specifically at vitamin K dependent factors, minimum hemostatic levels have been reported as 20-40% for factor II, 25-30% for factor IX, and 10-20% for factors VII and X (82)(90). Studies on patients with congenital multiple factor deficiencies (such as congenital Factor V and Factor VII deficiency "F5F8D" and congenital deficiency of Vitamin K-dependent clotting factors "VKCFD1") indicate bleeding tendencies are of the same magnitude as those in patients with isolated factor V or factor VII deficiency: this implies multiple deficiencies do not have an additive effect on bleeding risk (76). This is important as multiple factor deficiencies are usually encountered clinically and in addition it has been shown that prolongation of aPTT and PT is significantly greater if there are multiple deficiencies of various clotting factors, and this will occur at levels well above 75% (91). This in part explains the poor correlation of these tests with bleeding risk. Gulati et al., (84) analyzed factor levels in 83 patients on warfarin therapy with INR values ranging from 1.0 to 8.36: They found mean activity levels to be near or above 50% for II, VII, IX and X when the INR was less than 1.5 and that these did not fall below the hemostatic range until INR reached 2.5 (see Figure 2).

Surgery and Critical Care

In a study in neurosurgical patients, Matevosyan et al., (83) found PT values ranging from 12.8 -17.6 seconds (INR 1.3 - 1.7) but in all patients levels of factor II, VII and VIII were above 25% and most above 50% (median (range) for factor II 73% [40-107], factor VII 64% (25-124) and factor VIII 118% [43-547]. Chowdhury et al., (73) measured coagulation factor levels pre and post FFP infusion in critically-ill patients where reasons for prolonged PT and INR were multi-factorial, and found nearly 50% of patients with an INR >1.5 had factor levels above 30iu/dl and hence adequate for hemostasis.

Collins et al., (71) looked at coagulation factor levels in 38 patients with severe sepsis and abnormal coagulation tests. Mean levels of factors II, V, VII, X and XII were lower when compared to controls but only 21% of patients had one or more factor levels below the hemostatic threshold. In addition it is a frequent finding in hospitalized patients that levels of factor VIII and fibrinogen are supra normal (73, 83, 92). Collectively, the evidence from these studies is that over a range of clinical settings, coagulation factor levels are usually adequate for hemostasis at INR < 1.8 x control. Indeed the available data does not support the need to transfuse pre-procedural FFP in patients with mild coagulopathy, defined as an INR $\leq$ 2.0.

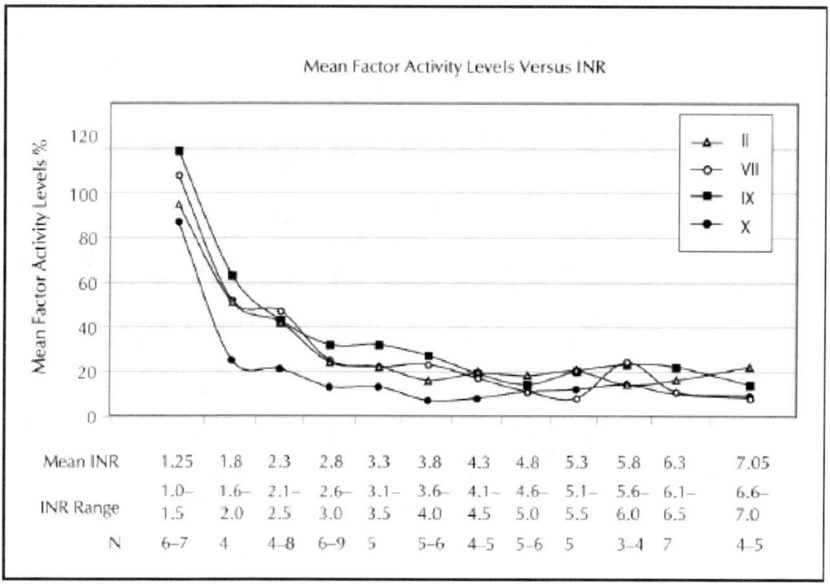

Figure 2. A side by side comparison of mean factor activity levels versus International Normalized Ratio (INR) in 83 patients taking warfarin (INR range 1.0-8.26). Taken from Gulati G, Hevelow M, George M, Behling E, Siegel J(84).

Liver Disease

The liver produces almost all procoagulants exclusively (except for factor VIII and von Willebrand factor) and consequently the INR has become a surrogate marker for liver failure, and is used in scoring systems such as the MELD and UKELD. Deitcher (93) found the INR in liver disease did not reflect the same degree of deficiencies of the same coagulation factors as in patients on warfarin therapy. For any given INR, the degree of factor V and

VII deficiency may be greater in liver disease but the opposite may be true for Factor X. In this study, over an INR range of 1.3 to 1.9, mean factor levels ranged from 31-65% (factor II), 40-70% (factor V) and 22-60% (factor VII). All these levels would be considered adequate for hemostasis. These studies mirror findings from decades ago where Manucci et al., (94) reported factor levels of over 30iu/dl for all of the studied 15 patients undergoing liver biopsy with a prolonged PT. There is also a larger variation in INR values in liver disease relative to the sensitivity of thromboplastin reagent used. Kovacs et al., (95) found that by using different thromboplastin reagents, the INR value in a cirrhotic patient could vary from 1.76 to 2.39. This is clinically important as the INR is used in scoring systems of liver disease and hence in prioritization of patients for liver transplant (78).

It is becoming clear that an INR of 1.6 in a stable cirrhotic patient does not reflect the same bleeding (or thrombotic) risk as in a warfarinized patient, a septic patient with low grade DIC, a patient with traumatic brain injury or a patient undergoing cardiac bypass (96). There are profound local and systemic differences in such coagulopathies. This is quite simply because even if the level of pro-coagulant factors are similar in each setting (resulting in similar PT, INR or aPTT), these tests do not consider activity of tissue factor, natural anticoagulants, ongoing fibrinolysis, platelet activation/consumption, endothelial involvement and an under-estimated degree of cross-trafficking between coagulation and inflammatory molecules (97). The cell-based model of hemostasis (98), as opposed to the traditional description of intrinsic and extrinsic pathways takes this more into account. In sepsis (71) and liver disease (99), a fall in pro-coagulation factors leading to a raised PT/INR is usually accompanied by a concurrent fall in anticoagulants like protein C and antithrombin with preserved thrombin generation. In addition, there is a rise in acute phase proteins like fibrinogen and factor VIII due to constant endothelial activation. This "re-balancing" of coagulation factors often means patients are not at increased risk of bleeding and in fact there is a significant thrombosis rate in such patients (100, 101). All coagulation test abnormalities must be evaluated within a clinical context, and using a single threshold INR that can apply to all patients is possibly the wrong approach, and indeed many guidelines now use different (higher) thresholds for patients with liver disease (see table 1).

4c. Evidence that Conventional Doses of FFP Correct Mild to Moderately Prolonged PT-INR Values

Although there is little hard evidence that a mild to moderate prolongation of PT/ INR is associated with a significantly increased risk of bleeding, the basis of transfusing prophylactic FFP is on the premise that it will correct the PT/INR to a value of <1.5 and so reduce the associated (perceived) risk. However, a multitude of studies have demonstrated that conventional doses of FFP rarely correct these mild abnormalities (1, 8, 38). Studies show that in patients with mildly prolonged clotting times, over a range of clinical settings, including liver biopsy and critical care, only 10-23% of patients will experience adequate correction following FFP transfusion (1, 8, 14, 94, 102-105). In the recent National Audit of FFP transfusion in England and Wales (1) across nearly 5000 transfusions, the median INR correction was only 0.2-0.3 depending on the INR. Another larger study in the US looked at over 70,000 plasma transfusions in 10 institutions, and found a median change in INR of 0.2 with 25% of transfusions resulting in no change or even an increase in INR (8). In a multi-center observational study in critical care, again the median change in PT or INR taken 6 hours post transfusion in 276 patients was minimal and greater with a higher pre-transfusion INR (median change -0.1, -0.4, -1.0, -2.5 for pre transfusion INRs in ranges <1.5, 1.6-2.5, 2.6-3.5, and >3.5 respectively) (17). Abdel-Wahab et al., (102) prospectively evaluated the effects of plasma on PT/INR in 121 hospital patients with pre-transfusion PT between 13.1-17 seconds. Less than 1% of patients experienced full correction and only 15% corrected half way to normal, most of whom received one to two units of FFP.

What has become clearer with these studies is that higher INR values (and hence lower coagulation factor levels or more severe coagulopathies) correct more profoundly with FFP. Holland & Brooks (38, 106) reported the effect of FFP on INR values in 179 patients in a retrospective study which excluded trauma and patients in the operating room (see Figure 3). Their data indicated that only at an INR of ≥1.8 that patients can be expected to experience a significant post-transfusion reduction in their INR. In addition, with an INR of ≤1.7, factor levels are usually > 30% and adequate for hemostasis. Similar graphs and findings have been reproduced in other studies (8, 17, 107). At lower levels of INR (1.3 -1.8) only very small changes in clotting factor activity will occur for a given volume of FFP compared to much more significant increases when the INR >2.5. One reason for this relationship between FFP and INR is the INR of FFP itself which can range from 0.9 to 1.4

(106) due heterogeneity between units derived from different donors. In addition, there are the effects of dilution with citrate and loss of factors incurred by thawing and delays in transfusion.

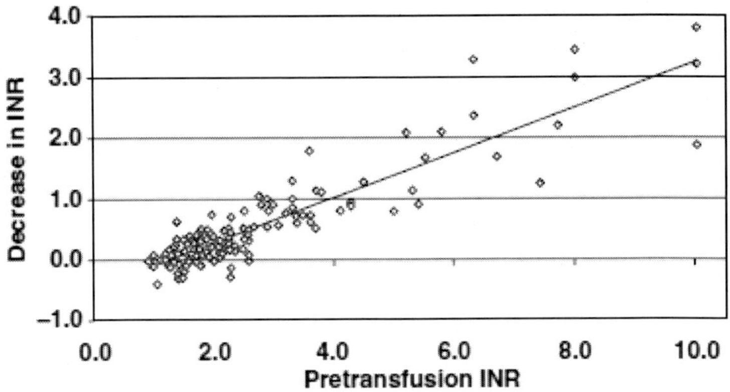

Figure 3a. The linear relationship between pre-transfusion INR and the decrease in INR per 500ml-unit of FFP in adult patients.

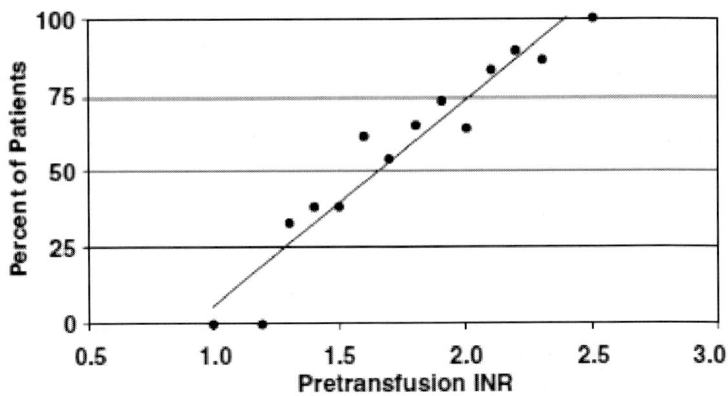

Figure 3b. Percentage of patients experiencing a significant change in INR following FFP transfusion in adult patients. Both taken from Holland LL and Brooks JP(38).

It has become clear that conventional doses of FFP will not correct mildly prolonged PT (less than 17 seconds) or INR (less than 1.8 x control) values. Most guidelines recommend a prophylactic dose of 10-15ml/kg (see Table 1) and studies indicate that doses actually given are often less or that a blanket approach of two to four units is used, particularly in prophylactic transfusion (8, 17). For example, a retrospective study of 70000 plasma transfusions found that over 75% of transfusions were equal/less than 12mls/kg and that 62% of transfusions consisted of one or two units(8). It is unclear where the recommended dose of 10-15mls/kg comes from but possibly from a trial in 1968 looking at risk of intracranial hemorrhage in neonates with a "thrombotest" of less than 10% (108): Neonates who received 10mls/kg FFP did have reduced risk of death but no data was shown to confirm the assertion that a dose of 10mls/kg corrected the thrombotest. Typically transfusion of one unit per kg of a coagulation factor raises its level by 1%. It follows that conventional doses of 10-15 mls/kg of FFP will only raise levels by 10-15% and indeed studies, many in patients undergoing liver biopsy (94, 109), show that on average FFP transfusions (8-12ml/kg) increased factor levels only by around 10iu/dl. Muller et al., (110) measured factor levels, thrombin generation and viscoelastographic parameters in 38 non-bleeding critically ill patients before and after 12ml/kg FFP transfusion: They also found factor levels increased by around 10% after FFP transfusion but still remained at the lower end of the normal range and that thrombin generation and viscoelastographic parameters were largely unchanged.

Makris et al., (90) showed that in warfarin-treated patients, giving roughly 12mls/kg FFP (or 800mls FFP) raised factors II, VII, IX and X by only 9 -14 iu/dl. Chowdhury et al., (73) in their study on 22 critically-ill patients, found a volume of 12mls/kg FFP did not significantly increment factors V, VIII, IX or X, and that 30mls/kg are required to reliably correct the INR and adequately increment factor levels.. Importantly the volume of FFP required depends not just on the initial INR, but also the target INR; the difference in volume between a goal of an INR of 1.3 and a goal INR of 1.7 is two liters of FFP at all initial INR values (38). Most guidelines do not specify any dose-adjustment based on initial and target values.

4d. Challenges for Trials Evaluating Prophylactic FFP Transfusion and Clinical Outcomes

The call for RCTs looking at bleeding complications in patients receiving prophylactic FFP transfusions has never been greater and voiced repeatedly in the literature (69, 105, 111-113). A recent Cochrane review failed to identify any randomized clinical trials (out of 843 screened) that assessed the effects of liberal and restrictive thresholds of at least one coagulation test used to guide FFP transfusion in critically ill patients (114). Attempts to carry out large RCTs have been abandoned in the past: The Study of Hemostasis in Invasive

Procedures trial (SHIP) (13) was to involve 16 sites and 1,300 participants undergoing invasive hepatic procedures with a pre-procedure INR of 1.3 to 1.9, randomly assigned to plasma or no treatment. It was terminated due to difficulty identifying suitable elective patients. A multi-center open label RCT comparing prophylactic 12ml/kg FFP transfusion to no FFP transfusion in critically-ill patients with an INR in between 1.5 and 3 undergoing an invasive procedure (Transfusion of FFP in non-bleeding ICU patients-TOPIC) also prematurely terminated due to slow inclusion (14). Of the 81 patients randomized in TOPIC, bleeding outcomes were no different between transfused and non-transfused groups. Duration of mechanical ventilation, and incidence of ventilator-associated pneumonia were higher in the transfused group which agrees with other retrospective studies in critical care (61). There was a trend to higher mortality in the non-transfused but this group also had an increased prevalence of liver disease, which was an independent predictor of mortality.

The authors have highlighted the challenges faced in successfully carrying out such trials: Firstly there is a high rate of declined consent as would be expected in critical care and this was 25% in TOPIC: Deferred proxy consent has been suggested to deal with consent issues in emergency and critical care (115). Secondly, clinicians have strong-held beliefs about prophylactic plasma transfusion: A survey carried out after termination of the TOPIC trial showed that almost all clinicians felt the trial was ethically justified and well-designed with clinically relevant outcomes (113). Yet less than half stated the trial was widely supported in their department and more than half felt that certain patient groups should be excluded from the trial. It seems another important barrier to patient inclusion is physician-driven and this is bidirectional; Physicians excluded patients when they felt risk of bleeding was high and they did not want to risk randomization to omission of FFP transfusion but they mainly excluded patients because of concerns about fluid overload and risks of TACO and TRALI if randomized to FFP transfusion. In keeping with this, a RCT looking at bleeding events with and without prophylactic plasma transfusion prior to percutaneous tracheostomy in ICU prematurely terminated as the occurrence of bleeding was so rare in either group that physicians were unwilling to risk randomization to plasma transfusion (116). Lack of knowledge regarding FFP dosage is also a problem. 30% of physicians felt 12mls/kg was too high a dose in the TOPIC trial although this is the lower limit of what is stated in most guidelines and actually nowhere near the 35mls/kg that may be required to correct mildly prolonged PT/INR values (73). It is clear that in order to address these issues, pre-trial questioning and education of physicians about transfusion indications, dosing and effects is necessary for successful inclusion into trials (113). It has been demonstrated that beliefs about FFP are amenable to change, and education of physicians has been shown to reduce inappropriate FFP use (117)(118) Behavioral interventions such as educational campaigns, prospective audits, and request forms with guidelines printed on them have all been shown to be effective (119-122). In line with this, Matesyovan et al., (83) report an impressive 75% reduction in plasma transfusion after implementation of modified FFP guidelines for neurosurgical patients.

Another challenge in these studies is the choice of primary outcome: Bleeding *per se* is subjective and outcomes need to take into account not only the volume but also its locality, the hemodynamic response to bleeding and the need for red blood cell transfusions (114). Recommendations for potential meaningful clinical end-points of hemostasis have been suggested by Levy and colleagues (96). Different bleeding tools have been validated in different populations: the HEME tool used in the TOPIC trial is well validated in ICU patients but the WHO bleeding scale is validated more in cancer patients. Finally, hemostatic control is itself only a surrogate marker of mortality and so studies need to measure mortality in addition as an outcome (123).

5. The Role of Global Assays in Guiding Prophylactic FFP Transfusion

Most recent guidelines agree that currently the best available predictor of bleeding remains a structured personal and family history of bleeding diatheses with physical examination (88, 124). This is probably reassuring enough for clinicians looking after well and/or uncomplicated patients having minor procedures. However until validated alternatives to conventional coagulation tests become widely available, or well conducted trials are successfully completed, prophylactic correction will probably continue to be practiced in patients with co-morbidities such as liver disease or critical illness and/or in patients having procedures with a moderate to high risk of bleeding.

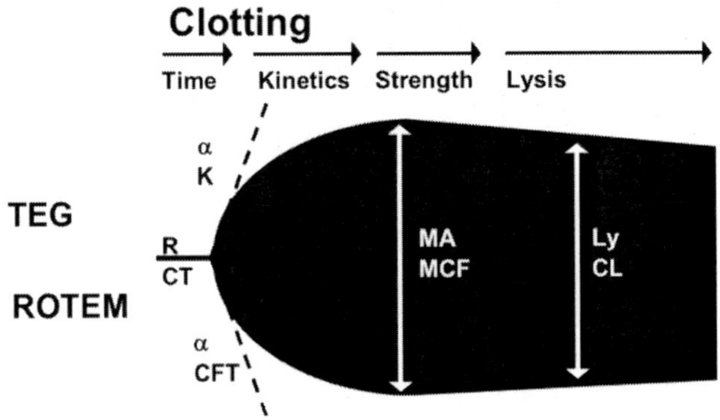

Figure 4a. Schematic TEG (upper trace) / ROTEM (lower trace) traces showing common parameters: reaction (R) time/ Clotting time (CT), Clot Formation Time (k/CFT), alpha angle (α), Maximum Amplitude (MA)/Maximum Clot Firmness (MCF) and Lysis (Ly)/Clot Lysis (CL). Taken from Johansson PI, Stissing T, Bochsen L, Ostrowski SR(125).

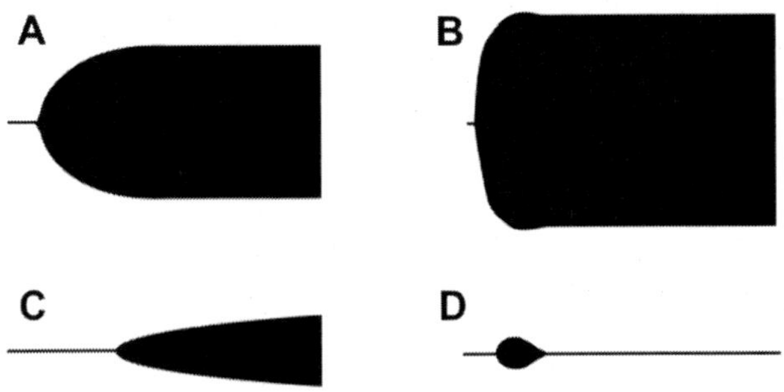

Figure 4b. Schematic presentation of various abnormal viscoelastic tracings. A) Normal B) Hypercoagability C) Hypocoagulopathy D) Primary Hyperfibrinolysis. Taken from Johansson PI, Stissing T, Bochsen L, Ostrowski SR(125).

Viscoelastography (VET) is a point of care (POC) test that is a dynamic global test of hemostasis with a more rapid turn-around time than conventional coagulation tests. There are two commercially available devices, both based on the original invention of Hartert in 1948 the Thromboelastogram or TEG® (Hemoscope, USA) and rotational elastometry or ROTEM® (Pentapharma, Munich, Germany). Details can be found in the literature (126, 127). In both tests, the rate of polymerization and overall clot strength is displayed visually and numerically on a trace and provides a dynamic assessment of the process of clot initiation, formation, stability, and dissolution (see Figure 4) as described in the cell-based model of coagulation [89]. VETs have become widely used in orthoptic liver transplantation (OLT) (128, 129), cardiac surgery (130-132), trauma (125, 133, 134) and obstetrics (135) in order to diagnose the causes of established bleeding and allow timely focused interventions. They may also be useful in identifying and monitoring hemophiliac patients (136, 137) and other rare bleeding disorders (138). Systematic reviews in trauma, liver transplantation and cardiac surgery do show that VETs decrease transfusion of blood products (139-141) but these studies were not powered to look at outcome or mortality.

A RCT of VETs versus conventional tests to guide transfusion of FFP in liver transplantation, demonstrated a significant reduction in FFP in the group managed with VET (142), however, there is currently little information regarding the use of VET to on guide prophylactic FFP transfusions in these settings. Pietri et al., (143) have yet to publish their RCT looking at cirrhotic patients having invasive procedures with either prolonged PT-INR and/or thrombocytopenia. Patients are randomized to either TEG®- or conventional coagulation test-based care and initial results show far fewer prophylactic blood product transfusion in the TEG® group with no bleeding complications. This is in-keeping with the fact that cirrhotic patients often have coagulation test values that suggest a bleeding tendency with prolonged PT/INR and low platelet values, but VETs and thrombin generation assays often indicate a normal or even hyper-coaguable hemostatic profile, and indeed an increasing number of these patients are able to undergo major surgery, such as liver transplantation without the need for FFP and platelet transfusions (144-146).

Guidelines published by the European Society of Anaesthesiology on management of peri-operative bleeding state there is currently no evidence for VETs as predictors of bleeding but base this statement on four studies in cardiac surgery (147). The French Society of Anaesthesia and Intensive Care have released a similar statement in their guidelines (124) but refer to one paediatric study using a non-VET test of platelet inhibition. However, VETs may be better placed to predict global risk of bleeding than conventional tests, as they reflect pro- and anti-coagulant activity, the contribution of cellular components to clot formation, total thrombin generation and fibrin breakdown (125). To date there are only small prospective studies assessing VETs as predictors of bleeding in non-bleeding patients, and these have conflicting results (148-153). Such studies are too small and heterogeneous with high risks of bias, but in those studies where VETs were shown to be useful predictors, the parameters that look at speed of clot strengthening (alpha angle/Clot Formation Time (CFT) and k value) rather than time to initial clot formation (R time/ Clotting Time (CT)) appear more relevant to bleeding risk.

This would explain the poor correlation of PT and INR with bleeding risk as these tests reflect initiation more than clot kinetics or ultimate clot strength. In sepsis-associated coagulopathy (71) and liver disease (144) it has been shown that although activation of coagulation is delayed (probably reflecting lower levels of pro-coagulants such as factor II, VII and X), thrombin generation is normal or even enhanced despite prolonged PT/INR values and/or low platelet counts. In their prospective observational study of 58 trauma patients Park M.S et al., (154) describe accelerated rate of clot formation (alpha angle) and maximum clot strength (MA) as well as low levels of anticoagulants like protein C and high fibrinogen counts: these all suggest a hyper-coaguable environment which is supported by the high thromboembolic rate in trauma patients despite these same patients having prolonged aPTT and PT values. Varying correlations between PT/INR and the R time/CT and similarly between MA/MCF and platelet count and/or fibrinogen level have been described (144, 155, 156). This variability can be partly explained by different activators and different specimens. However a crucial difference is that conventional tests reflect isolated pathways in clot formation and VETs reflect the balance of both pro- and anti-coagulants and how they all interact with platelets and other blood cells as VETs are done in whole blood. In addition the R time or CT only prolong once factor concentrations dip to 20-30% of normal (157-159) and therefore are less sensitive to PT or INR elevations ≤ 1.7 x control. They may therefore be a better reflection of true bleeding potential than conventional tests and we should more reassured by a lack of, not presence of, a significant correlation between VET parameters and aPTT, PT and INR. This highlights the problem that there is no gold standard test to compare VETs with when assessing bleeding risk. Other challenges in validating VETs include the lack of standardization within and between TEG® and ROTEM® systems (160, 161) as well as lack of definitions for hypo-and hyper-coaguability (162).

6. Evidence for Prophylactic FFP in Specific Clinical Scenarios

6a. Liver Disease

A large proportion of prophylactic FFP is given to patients with liver disease. A national audit of blood product use over 1300 cases of cirrhosis reported that 76% of patients receiving prophylactic FFP received it prior to a procedure and that 47% of these patients had an INR ≤ 2.0 (24). There is now a significant volume of evidence in patients with liver disease that PT, aPTT and INR do not correlate with bleeding risk and that FFP does little to attenuate this risk (163, 164). Specifically looking at liver biopsies, Ewe et al., (165) were the first to observe bleeding times after percutaneous laparoscopic liver biopsy in 200 patients and correlate this to coagulation indices including platelet count. They found no correlation and that the few cases of prolonged bleeding stopped with compression alone if necessary. Gilmore et al., *(166)* looked at 1500 liver biopsies in England and Wales; and found that of the patients that bled, 89.6% had an INR <1.3, however, the incidence of bleeding increased from 3.3% to 7.1% if INR was ≥1.5. Several studies since (one looking at over 9000 biopsies (167)),have failed to show a link between hemorrhage and abnormal clotting profiles after liver biopsy (75, 165, 167, 168). Youssef et al., (103) carried out a split retrospective-prospective study in patients with Child-Pugh Class B and C liver disease who received FFP transfusions and only 10-12% of patients achieved the target PT. In their recent systematic review Yang et al., (11) identified seven RCTs addressing prophylactic FFP use in liver disease for a variety indications and outcomes including laboratory correction of coagulopathy (94) and prevention of veno-occlusive disease after stem cell transplantation(169). No significant benefit across all outcomes was reported. It is also becoming more common practice to perform orthotoptic liver transplantation without FFP(146, 170), as most centers will only transfuse FFP if there is active bleeding, and avoid prophylactic FFP as the excess volume increases portal hypertension, and paradoxically will increase blood loss (171).

The finding of a prolonged PT ratio or INR is common simply because these tests reflect pro coagulant levels that are usually decreased in liver disease. There is a “re-balancing” of hemostasis in stable chronic liver disease (99, 172) and patients may not even be vitamin K-deficient as is often assumed (76). Primary hemostasis is relatively preserved and the concentrations of both pro- and anticoagulant factors are both decreased in liver disease (99). Hence, thrombin generation is actually normal (144) and may even be enhanced (173). It is of note that rather than there being lower rates of thromboembolic events, as would be presumed if these patients were indeed “auto-anticoagulated”, there is in fact a similar, or even increased thrombo-embolic rate in patients with cirrhotic and non-cirrhotic liver disease, and the role of pharmacological thrombo-prophylaxis is now being discussed despite prolonged PT-INR values (100, 101). Collectively this evidence supports the notion that plasma should not be administered to non-bleeding patients with liver disease and an INR ≤ 2 who are undergoing an invasive procedure. In addition, although more evidence is needed, VETs and thrombin generation assays may have better clinical utility in assessing hemorrhagic and thrombotic risk in these patients (145) and large scale clinical trials are urgently needed.

Although acute liver failure (ALF) is defined by a raised PT/INR, clinically significant bleeding is rare, and usually mucosal or superficial in nature (174). It has been found that most patients have normal hemostatic parameters on VETs with no correlation between INR in bleeders and non-bleeders (175). Of interest, hyper-coaguable parameters have been noted in ALF on TEG® in the presence of a systemic inflammatory response syndrome, raised lactate and phosphate, hyperammoneamia and encephalopathy (175). In a multi-variant analysis the single most important component determining clot strength in TEG® is the platelet count, followed by fibrinogen concentration and lastly pro-coagulant factor levels (175). Prophylactic administration of FFP simply to correct an abnormal INR is not justified in ALF and will obscure the value of INR as a dynamic indicator or worsening or improving liver function. One randomized trial compared prophylactic FFP transfusion with a control group of no FFP in paracetamol overdose (176). There were only 20 patients but no differences in clinical outcomes was shown. Concerns about coagulopathy arise prior to performing invasive procedures in ALF such as placement of intracranial pressure (ICP) monitors where small studies report success with recombinant factor VIIa (rFVIIa) (177-179). However the evidence as to its efficacy in reducing bleeding complications or for the optimal dose regime is poor as publications are limited to small case series, and there are concerns about the potential for thrombo-embolic complications. Indeed, efficacy has primarily been based on its ability to reverse the PT/INR, rather than on clinical outcomes. Evidence regarding the use of prothrombin complex concentrate (PCC) in a prophylactic role is lacking but similar concerns exist (180). Plasma exchange plasmapheresis with FFP may be beneficial in correcting INR and improving hemodynamics (181). Prior to invasive procedures in patients with ALF, fibrinogen levels <1g/l should be corrected with cryoprecipitate or fibrinogen concentrate and platelet count of 50000/uL is acceptable (182).

6b. Procedures in Critical Care

Central Venous Access

Central venous access is a commonplace procedure in most hospitals and measures to reduce complication rates include ultrasound-guidance and strict aseptic technique. It is still standard practice in many institutions to correct abnormal PT/INR values with prophylactic plasma despite the fact that studies fail to show a link between these profiles and bleeding episodes (183-187). Della Vigna et al., (187) found no bleeding complications when they retrospectively reviewed 122 CVC line insertions in cancer patients with prolonged PT/aPTT or low platelets. 37% of these patients actually had PT/APTT values >2.2 x normal and/or platelet count less than 50,000/ul. Weigand et al., (185) report no difference in hemoglobin decreases from 196 patients with and without abnormal PT or platelet counts. Doerfler et al., (188) report similar findings in a prospective study of 104 central line placements and found in the rare cases of superficial bleeding (6.5% of procedures), patients suffered more with severe thrombocytopenia (range 6000/uL to 37,000/uL) rather than abnormal PT and/or aPTT. Mumtaz et al., (183) also found bleeding was limited to the insertion site in the few patients who bled in their study of 330 line insertions, and that a platelet count of less than 50,000/uL was associated with a small risk of bleeding but prophylactic correction of PT was not. Another retrospective review of 490 critical care patients, found that in the rare cases of superficial bleeding, this appeared to be related to the experience of the physician rather than to defects in hemostasis (189). These studies all suggest a platelet count of > 30,000/uL and skill level of the operator are the main determinants of bleeding, not the raised PT/INR, indicating that prophylactic correction with FFP of mildly elevated PT/INR is unlikely to be of benefit, but may be harmful if it results in TRALI or TACO.

Tracheostomy

Veelo et al., (116) report the findings of a small RCT where 35 critically ill patients having percutaneous tracheostomy either with a thrombocytopenia (40-100,000/uL), prolonged PT (14.7-20 seconds), or treatment with acetylsalicylic acid were randomized to correction or no correction with blood products. Not only was the incidence of bleeding very low leading to resistance from physicians to correct values (ultimately prematurely terminating the trial), but correction of PT with FFP was marginal (mean decrease 0.4 seconds +/- 0.56), in keeping with numerous other studies, and there was no difference in median blood loss between the "correction" and "no correction" groups. Again operator experience and technique have a greater bearing and using multiple or single step dilator techniques may be associated with lower bleeding risk (190, 191)[183, 184].

Thoracocentesis

Over 20 years ago, McVay and Toy (74) retrospectively reviewed 217 patients undergoing thoracocentesis with variable use of ultrasound and operator experience and found no difference in bleeding complications between those with normal and abnormal aPTT or PT values (up to 2.0 x normal) or mild (50-99,000/uL) to moderate (25-49,000/uL) thrombocytopenia. In another retrospective study of 100 patients with malignant pleural effusions, hemothorax complicated thoracocentesis in two patients but none had abnormal clotting profiles (192). Hibbert et al., (193) retrospectively looked at over 1000 episodes of thoracocentesis and found the incidence of hemorrhagic complications to be very low (0.4%) and all four complications occurred in the group of patients given either pre-procedural platelets or plasma. In a retrospective analysis of 1076 ultrasound-guided thoracocenteses, no bleeding complications were observed and pre-procedure INR exceeded 2.0 in 139 cases and exceeded 3.0 in 32 cases (194). Finally Puchalski et al., (195) prospectively observed 312 thoracocenteses where 42% of patients had at least one risk factor for bleeding such as INR > 1.5 x control, platelet count < 50,000/uL, creatinine > 1.5mg/dl or use of clopidogrel or heparin: They found no difference in pre and post hematocrit levels between patients with and without one or more bleeding risk factors. A recent review of risk factors for bleeding following thoracocentesis concluded there was no evidence for correction of mildly elevated INR values or mild to moderate thrombocytopenia and that future studies should focus on patients with INR values 3-5 x control and platelet counts of 10-25,000/uL (196).

Overall, these studies suggest that pre-procedural (prophylactic) administration of FFP is unnecessary if the INR is ≤ 2.0, and will in any case have a very limited effect in terms of reducing the INR.

6c. Cardiac Surgery

Cardiac bypass brings with it unique coagulation disturbances including platelet dysfunction, hyperfibrinolysis, coagulation factor consumption and effects of anticoagulation. It has been common practice to prime bypass with FFP or to give FFP at the end of surgery irrespective of bleeding or coagulation indices although this practice is diminishing with the increasing use of VETs. One prospective randomized trial in 20 infants having cardiac bypass found a trend towards reduced blood product transfusion when FFP was used to prime the pump versus no FFP (197) but no difference in 24 hour blood loss. There are also randomized trials reporting reduced blood product transfusion and blood loss when acute preoperative plasmapheresis is used in cardiac surgery (198-200). A systematic review identified six RCTs involving 363 patients that compared FFP with either no FFP, a colloid-like substance, or packed red cells as a control arm either before during or after surgery: The authors commented on poor methodology and heterogeneity in the studies and could not find evidence for reduced 24 hour blood loss with FFP (201). A more recent meta-analysis of eight RCTs (11) also failed to show a difference in 24-hour blood loss between groups given prophylactic FFP and a control arm, (again be it no FFP, a colloid-like substance, or comparing different types of plasma). Overall Yang et al., (202) identified 15 trials which have evaluated prophylactic FFP in non-bleeding patients with cardiac disease and no consistent benefit could be demonstrated.

6d. Neurosurgical Procedures

In neurosurgery, the potential consequences of bleeding into a closed space are catastrophic and many clinicians aim to keep INR < 1.3 x control. A retrospective survey of ICP placement in severe head injury patients with INR of 1.3-1.6 x control showed no differences in bleeding complications with or without FFP and that transfused patients suffered significantly more delays in their procedure (mean 19.2 hours +/- 19.7 hours versus 8.8 +/- 13.9 hours, p < 0.002) (203). Several reviews (46, 204, 205) fail to support the use of FFP in a range of neurosurgical scenarios ranging from ICP monitor placement (where depth of monitor seems to play a larger role in bleeding) to traumatic brain injury (TBI). Of concern in TBI, there is an abundance of tissue factor leading to accelerated consumption of coagulant factors and platelets and possible further bleeding (204). Documented coagulopathy is highly variable ranging from 10 to 97.5% [196]. Some advocate the use of prophylactic FFP in severe TBI where Glasgow Coma Scale (GCS) is <6 but this has little evidence-base (46). In a double-blinded RCT comparing FFP with saline, death and delayed ICH were worse in the FFP group (206) and may have been caused by consequent raised intracranial pressures or even a pro-thrombotic effect of FFP with resultant vascular ischemia. Schramm et al., (207) reviewed 1211 neurosurgical patients over one year, 200 of whom had spinal surgery: Prolonged PT or INR was not associated with increased bleeding risk but the combination of prolonged aPTT with a bleeding history (not prolonged aPTT on its own) was. Matevosyan et al., (83) tested plasma from 25 neurosurgical patients with an INR of 1.3-1.7 for levels of factors II,VII and VIII. The median factor level was 57% (range 25 -124%). Based on these findings this group modified their plasma transfusion guidelines and reduced ordering of FFP for mildly prolonged INR in neurosurgical patients by 75%.

Overall these papers demonstrate that neurosurgical patients with mild prolongations of INR $\leq$ 1.8 x control have hemostatically normal levels of important coagulation factors and prophylactic plasma does not reduce bleeding risk and can lead to detrimental delay in treatment in TBI.

6e. Reversal of Warfarin Toxicity in the Absence of Bleeding

The majority of guidelines now recommend using PCCs rather than FFP for the urgent reversal of warfarin overdose or prior to emergency surgery (208). The efficacy and rapidity of INR reduction over vitamin K (209) and FFP (90) have been shown although prospective clinical trials comparing therapies are largely lacking. In one study, FFP was compared with PCC in cardiac bypass surgical patients with preoperative INR values of greater than 2.1 (210). There was a trend towards reduced 24-hour chest drain output in the PCC group and a trend towards increased fluid overload, transfusion requirement and ooziness in the FFP group, but mortality was not reported. Stanworth et al., (211) in their systematic review also identified smaller studies comparing conventional FFP with different formulations of pathogen-reduced FFP in warfarinized subjects but did not find any significant difference in laboratory or clinical outcomes. In summary, PCC corrects INR faster and more completely than FFP, which in turn corrects faster than vitamin K but it is unclear if this equates to equivalent reductions in bleeding risk. There is no high quality evidence to support transfusion of FFP or PCC *prophylactically* in warfarin overdose in the absence of bleeding. Most guidelines recommend merely withholding of warfarin or administration of vitamin K if risk of bleeding is deemed high or INR value is very high (above 8 x control) (208).

PCCs are sterile lyophilized concentrates of vitamin-K dependent coagulation factors containing factor II, VII, IX and X and a variable amount of factor VII. PCCs are rapid to mix and administer, avoid volume overload (as little as 60mls necessary), avoid the risks of TRALI, and produce reproducible and predictable augmentation in coagulation factors (212). Many patients on warfarin therapy are elderly with co-existing cardiac problems, and use of PCC avoids the inevitable volume overload and dilutional problems that accompany FFP administration. The main concerns are cost and an unclear thrombotic risk. The recent addition of anticoagulants and small amounts of heparin to PCC formulations may well have reduced the thrombotic risk [117]. It has been demonstrated that in trauma patients receiving PCC, compared to those that did not, endogenous thrombin potential is increased for several days post operatively, and also that antithrombin (AT) levels remain low, implying a potential pro-thrombotic state not reflected by standard coagulation tests (213). It took a number of years before the increased risk of arterial thrombo-embolic events associated with the use of rFVIIa was recognized, another drug that acts by enhancing thrombin generation (214).

In summary there is a decreasing role for FFP in warfarin reversal as PCC is preferred in emergencies or in bleeding patients, and vitamin K or withholding of warfarin is effective in stable non-bleeding patients or the elective setting.

Overcoming some of these problems will require new, and more novel ways of designing these clinical trials, such as large-scale cohort studies. However, summating all the available evidence to date, it is now clear that the practice of giving FFP in order to reduce a perceived bleeding risk is of little or no benefit in stable patients with mild prolongation of PT/INR, and may in fact be harmful. It is time to move to a much more restrictive, and evidence based practice when transfusing FFP.

Conclusion

There is currently no high quality evidence to support prophylactic FFP transfusion to correct PT or INR values $\leq$ 1.8 x control in non-bleeding patients across all ranges of specialties. There is also a lack of confidence in current guidelines for both prophylactic and therapeutic FFP use and high levels of inappropriate use worldwide (up to 80%). Conventional coagulation tests such as PT and INR do not accurately indicate bleeding risk and need to be interpreted within their clinical context. Global assays such as viscoelastography may be more useful, but more evidence is needed supported by large-scale clinical trials. In liver disease, many patients VETs show preserved or enhanced thrombin generation when conventional tests suggest hypercoagulability and many guidelines now use higher threshold INR values of ≥ 2.0 x control in these patients. Standard doses of FFP (10-15mls/Kg) do not adequately correct PT or INR values less than 1.8 x control, and indeed coagulation factor levels, are, in most cases, above the hemostatic threshold of 30% in these patients. It is clear that standard doses of FFP are only effective in correcting profound coagulopathies and physicians need more education about the indications and dosing of FFP as this has been shown to have an impact on practice. RCTs looking at bleeding outcomes and mortality after prophylactic FFP transfusion have been terminated in the past due to challenges in recruiting patients, and resistance from physicians to expose patients to the risks FFP transfusion when bleeding risk is perceived to be low and resistance to expose patients to omission of FFP transfusion when the risk of bleeding is perceived to be high. In addition, bleeding outcomes are variable amongst studies looking at prophylactic FFP and the use of validated tools that incorporate bleeding volume, location, transfusion needs and mortality needs to be promoted. Future studies also need to include mandatory reporting of adverse effects of FFP such as ALI, circulatory overload, thrombosis and infection rates as well as delays incurred in performing procedures. Overcoming some of these problems will require new, and more novel ways of designing these clinical trials, such as large-scale cohort studies. However, summating all the available evidence to date, it is now clear that the practice of giving FFP in order to reduce a perceived bleeding risk is of little or no benefit in stable patients with mild prolongation of PT/INR, and may in fact be harmful. It is time to move to a much more restrictive, and evidence based practice when transfusing FFP.

References

[1] Stanworth SJ, Grant-Casey J, Lowe D, Laffan M, New H, Murphy MF, et al. The use of fresh-frozen plasma in England: high levels of inappropriate use in adults and children. *Transfusion.* 2011 Jan;51(1):62-70.

[2] Puetz J, Witmer C, Huang YS, Raffini L. Widespread use of fresh frozen plasma in US children's hospitals despite limited evidence demonstrating a beneficial effect. *J Pediatr.* 2012 Feb;160(2):210-5 e1.

[3] Sperry JL, Ochoa JB, Gunn SR, Alarcon LH, Minei JP, Cuschieri J, et al. An FFP:PRBC transfusion ratio >/=1:1.5 is associated with a lower risk of mortality after massive transfusion. *J Trauma.* 2008 Nov;65(5):986-93.

[4] Godier A, Ozier Y, Susen S. [1/1 plasma to red blood cell ratio: an evidence-based practice?]. *Ann Fr Anesth Reanim.* 2011 May;30(5):421-8.

[5] Greer SE, Rhynhart KK, Gupta R, Corwin HL. New developments in massive transfusion in trauma. *Curr Opin Anaesthesiol.* 2010 Apr;23(2):246-50.

[6] Dzik W, Rao A. Why do physicians request fresh frozen plasma? *Transfusion.* 2004 Sep;44(9):1393-4.

[7] Vlaar AP, in der Maur AL, Binnekade JM, Schultz MJ, Juffermans NP. A survey of physicians' reasons to transfuse plasma and platelets in the critically ill: a prospective single-centre cohort study. *Transfus Med.* 2009 Aug;19(4):207-12.

[8] Triulzi D, Gottschall J, Murphy E, Wu Y, Ness P, Kor D, et al. A multicenter study of plasma use in the United States. *Transfusion.* 2014 Dec 19.

[9] Roback JD, Caldwell S, Carson J, Davenport R, Drew MJ, Eder A, et al. Evidence-based practice guidelines for plasma transfusion. *Transfusion.* 2010 Jun;50(6):1227-39.

[10] Iorio A, Basileo M, Marchesini E, Materazzi M, Marchesi M, Esposito A, et al. The good use of plasma. A critical analysis of five international guidelines. *Blood Transfus.* 2008 Jan;6(1):18-24.

[11] Yang L, Stanworth S, Hopewell S, Doree C, Murphy M. Is fresh-frozen plasma clinically effective? An update of a systematic review of randomized controlled trials. *Transfusion.* [Review]. 2012 Aug;52(8):1673-86; quiz

[12] Triulzi DJ. The art of plasma transfusion therapy. *Transfusion.* 2006 Aug;46(8):1268-70.

[13] Dzik WH. The NHLBI Clinical Trials Network in transfusion medicine and hemostasis: an overview. *J Clin Apher.* 2006 Apr;21(1):57-9.

[14] Muller MC, Arbous MS, Spoelstra-de Man AM, Vink R, Karakus A, Straat M, et al. Transfusion of fresh-frozen plasma in critically ill patients with a coagulopathy before invasive procedures: a randomized clinical trial (CME). *Transfusion.* [Research Support, Non-U.S. Gov't]. 2015 Jan;55(1):26-35; quiz 25.

[15] Holland L, Sarode R. Should plasma be transfused prophylactically before invasive procedures? *Curr Opin Hematol.* 2006 Nov;13(6):447-51.

[16] Kor DJ, Stubbs JR, Gajic O. Perioperative coagulation management--fresh frozen plasma. *Best Pract Res Clin Anaesthesiol.* 2010 Mar;24(1):51-64.

[17] Stanworth SJ, Walsh TS, Prescott RJ, Lee RJ, Watson DM, Wyncoll D. A national study of plasma use in critical care: clinical indications, dose and effect on prothrombin time. *Crit Care.* 2011;15(2):R108.

[18] Tinmouth A, Thompson T, Arnold DM, Callum JL, Gagliardi K, Lauzon D, et al. Utilization of frozen plasma in Ontario: a provincewide audit reveals a high rate of inappropriate transfusions. *Transfusion.* [Research Support, Non-U.S. Gov't]. 2013 Oct;53(10):2222-9.

[19] Luk C, Eckert KM, Barr RM, Chin-Yee IH. Prospective audit of the use of fresh-frozen plasma, based on Canadian Medical Association transfusion guidelines. *CMAJ.* 2002 Jun 11;166(12):1539-40.

[20] Lauzier F, Cook D, Griffith L, Upton J, Crowther M. Fresh frozen plasma transfusion in critically ill patients. *Crit Care Med.* 2007 Jul;35(7):1655-9.

[21] Beloeil H, Brosseau M, Benhamou D. [Transfusion of fresh frozen plasma (FFP): audit of prescriptions]. *Ann Fr Anesth Reanim.* 2001 Oct;20(8):686-92.

[22] Pita-Ramirez L, Cabrera Carbajal BE, Ortega Zavala C. [Reasons for fresh frozen plasma transfusion in a general hospital]. *Rev Invest Clin.* 1999 Mar-Apr;51(2):89-92.

[23] Moiz B, Arif FM, Hashmi KZ. Appropriate and inappropriate use of fresh frozen plasma. *J Pak Med Assoc.* 2006 Aug;56(8):356-9.

[24] NHS Blood and Transplant. Multi Regional Audit of Blood Component use in patients with Cirrhosis 2014. http://hospitalbloodcouk/media/27102/10421-multi-regional-liver-audit-reportpdf (last accessed 5th April 2015).

[25] Benhamou D. The use of Fresh Frozen Plasma (FFP) in 2007 in France. *Transfus Clin Biol.* 2007 Dec;14(6):557-9.

[26] Gajic O, Dzik WH, Toy P. Fresh frozen plasma and platelet transfusion for nonbleeding patients in the intensive care unit: benefit or harm? *Crit Care Med.* 2006 May;34(5 Suppl):S170-3.

[27] O'Shaughnessy DF, Atterbury C, Bolton Maggs P, Murphy M, Thomas D, Yates S, et al. Guidelines for the use of fresh-frozen plasma,

cryoprecipitate and cryosupernatant. *Br J Haematol.* 2004 Jul;126(1):11-28.

[28] Practice guidelines for perioperative blood transfusion and adjuvant therapies: an updated report by the American Society of Anesthesiologists Task Force on Perioperative Blood Transfusion and Adjuvant Therapies. *Anesthesiology.* 2006 Jul;105(1):198-208.

[29] Grafstein E, Innes G. Guidelines for red blood cell and plasma transfusion for adults and children: an emergency physician's overview of the 1997 Canadian Blood Transfusion Guidelines. Part 2: Plasma transfusion and infectious risk. *J Emerg Med.* 1998 Mar-Apr;16(2):239-41.

[30] Clinical practice guidelines on the use of blood components. 2001 wwwNhmrcGovAu/_files_nhmrc/publications/attachments/cp78pdf (last accessed 5th April 2015).

[31] [Transfusion of fresh coagulated plasma: products, indications. General methods and recommendations]. *Transfus Clin Biol.* 2002 Nov-Dec;9(5-6):322-32.

[32] Heim MU, Hellstern P. [New cross-sectional guidelines of the German Medical Association for hemotherapy with fresh frozen plasma. Evidence-based recommendations for risk-benefit assessment]. *Anaesthesist.* 2010 Jan;59(1):80-5.

[33] Wong M, Droubatchevskaia N, Chipperfield Kate M, Wadsworth Louis D. Guidelines for frozen plasma transfusion. *British Columbia Medical Journal.* 2007;49(No. 6):9.

[34] Patel IJ, Davidson JC, Nikolic B, Salazar GM, Schwartzberg MS, Walker TG, et al. Consensus guidelines for periprocedural management of coagulation status and hemostasis risk in percutaneous image-guided interventions. *J Vasc Interv Radiol.* 2012 Jun;23(6):727-36.

[35] Westbrook A, Pettila V, Nichol A, Bailey MJ, Syres G, Murray L, et al. Transfusion practice and guidelines in Australian and New Zealand intensive care units. *Intensive Care Med.* 2010 Jul;36(7):1138-46.

[36] Hall DP, Lone NI, Watson DM, Stanworth SJ, Walsh TS. Factors associated with prophylactic plasma transfusion before vascular catheterization in non-bleeding critically ill adults with prolonged prothrombin time: a case-control study. *British journal of anaesthesia.* [Research Support, Non-U.S. Gov't]. 2012 Dec;109(6):919-27.

[37] Walsh TS, Stanworth SJ, Prescott RJ, Lee RJ, Watson DM, Wyncoll D. Prevalence, management, and outcomes of critically ill patients with

prothrombin time prolongation in United Kingdom intensive care units. *Crit Care Med.* 2010 Oct;38(10):1939-46.

[38] Holland LL, Brooks JP. Toward rational fresh frozen plasma transfusion: The effect of plasma transfusion on coagulation test results. *Am J Clin Pathol.* 2006 Jul;126(1):133-9.

[39] Shingina A, Barkun AN, Razzaghi A, Martel M, Bardou M, Gralnek I. Systematic review: the presenting international normalised ratio (INR) as a predictor of outcome in patients with upper nonvariceal gastrointestinal bleeding. *Aliment Pharmacol Ther.* 2011 May;33(9):1010-8.

[40] MacLennan S, Williamson LM. Risks of fresh frozen plasma and platelets. *J Trauma.* 2006 Jun;60(6 Suppl):S46-50.

[41] Agence francaise de sécurité sanitaire des produits de santé (Afssaps). Rapport annuel hémovigilance 2010. http://www.afssaps.fr/Activites/Hemovigilance/Hemovigilance/ (last accessed 26th march 20140

[42] Narick C, Triulzi DJ, Yazer MH. Transfusion-associated circulatory overload after plasma transfusion. *Transfusion.* 2011 Jul 18.

[43] Vlaar AP, Wortel K, Binnekade JM, van Oers MH, Beckers E, Gajic O, et al. The practice of reporting transfusion-related acute lung injury: a national survey among clinical and preclinical disciplines. *Transfusion.* 2010 Feb;50(2):443-51.

[44] Pinkerton PH, Callum JL. Rationalizing the clinical use of frozen plasma. *CMAJ.* 2010 Jul 13;182(10):1019-20.

[45] Pandey S, Vyas GN. Adverse effects of plasma transfusion. *Transfusion.* [Review]. 2012 May;52 Suppl 1:65S-79S.

[46] West KL, Adamson C, Hoffman M. Prophylactic correction of the international normalized ratio in neurosurgery: a brief review of a brief literature. *J Neurosurg.* 2011 Jan;114(1):9-18.

[47] Verghese SG. Elective fresh frozen plasma in the critically ill: what is the evidence? *Crit Care Resusc.* 2008 Sep;10(3):264-8.

[48] Khan H, Belsher J, Yilmaz M, Afessa B, Winters JL, Moore SB, et al. Fresh-frozen plasma and platelet transfusions are associated with development of acute lung injury in critically ill medical patients. *Chest.* 2007 May;131(5):1308-14.

[49] Popovsky MA. Transfusion-Related Acute Lung Injury: Incidence, Pathogenesis and the Role of Multicomponent Apheresis in Its Prevention. *Transfus Med Hemother.* 2008;35(2):76-9.

[50] Watson GA, Sperry JL, Rosengart MR, Minei JP, Harbrecht BG, Moore EE, et al. Fresh frozen plasma is independently associated with a higher

risk of multiple organ failure and acute respiratory distress syndrome. *J Trauma*. 2009 Aug;67(2):221-7; discussion 8-30.

[51] Hoffer A, Selman W. Transfusion. *J Neurosurg*. 2011 Jan;114(1):1; discussion 2.

[52] Buddeberg F, Schimmer BB, Spahn DR. Transfusion-transmissible infections and transfusion-related immunomodulation. *Best Pract Res Clin Anaesthesiol*. 2008 Sep;22(3):503-17.

[53] Sarani B, Dunkman WJ, Dean L, Sonnad S, Rohrbach JI, Gracias VH. Transfusion of fresh frozen plasma in critically ill surgical patients is associated with an increased risk of infection. *Critical care medicine*. [Research Support, Non-U.S. Gov't]. 2008 Apr;36(4):1114-8.

[54] Inaba K, Branco BC, Rhee P, Blackbourne LH, Holcomb JB, Teixeira PG, et al. Impact of plasma transfusion in trauma patients who do not require massive transfusion. *Journal of the American College of Surgeons*. 2010 Jun;210(6):957-65.

[55] Blajchman MA. Transfusion immunomodulation or TRIM: what does it mean clinically? *Hematology. 2005*;10 Suppl 1:208-14.

[56] Phan HH, Wisner DH. Should we increase the ratio of plasma/platelets to red blood cells in massive transfusion: what is the evidence? *Vox sanguinis*. [Review]. 2010 Apr;98(3 Pt 2):395-402.

[57] Rajasekhar A, Gowing R, Zarychanski R, Arnold DM, Lim W, Crowther MA, et al. Survival of trauma patients after massive red blood cell transfusion using a high or low red blood cell to plasma transfusion ratio. *Critical care medicine*. [Research Support, Non-U.S. Gov't Review]. 2011 Jun;39(6):1507-13.

[58] Spinella PC, Perkins JG, Grathwohl KW, Beekley AC, Niles SE, McLaughlin DF, et al. Effect of plasma and red blood cell transfusions on survival in patients with combat related traumatic injuries. *The Journal of trauma*. 2008 Feb;64(2 Suppl):S69-77; discussion S-8.

[59] Stainsby D, MacLennan S, Thomas D, Isaac J, Hamilton PJ. Guidelines on the management of massive blood loss. *Br J Haematol*. 2006 Dec;135(5):634-41.

[60] Eder AF, Herron RM, Jr., Strupp A, Dy B, White J, Notari EP, et al. Effective reduction of transfusion-related acute lung injury risk with male-predominant plasma strategy in the American Red Cross (2006-2008). *Transfusion*. 2010 Aug;50(8):1732-42.

[61] Dara SI, Rana R, Afessa B, Moore SB, Gajic O. Fresh frozen plasma transfusion in critically ill medical patients with coagulopathy. *Crit Care Med*. 2005 Nov;33(11):2667-71.

[62] Gajic O, Yilmaz M, Iscimen R, Kor DJ, Winters JL, Moore SB, et al. Transfusion from male-only versus female donors in critically ill recipients of high plasma volume components. *Crit Care Med.* 2007 Jul;35(7):1645-8.

[63] Toy P, Gajic O, Bacchetti P, Looney MR, Gropper MA, Hubmayr R, et al. Transfusion-related acute lung injury: incidence and risk factors. *Blood.* [Multicenter Study Research Support, N.I.H., Extramural]. 2012 Feb 16;119(7):1757-67.

[64] Chapman CE, Stainsby D, Jones H, Love E, Massey E, Win N, et al. Ten years of hemovigilance reports of transfusion-related acute lung injury in the United Kingdom and the impact of preferential use of male donor plasma. *Transfusion.* 2009 Mar;49(3):440-52.

[65] Li G, Rachmale S, Kojicic M, Shahjehan K, Malinchoc M, Kor DJ, et al. Incidence and transfusion risk factors for transfusion-associated circulatory overload among medical intensive care unit patients. *Transfusion.* 2011 Feb;51(2):338-43.

[66] Bolton-Maggs PH, Cohen H. Serious Hazards of Transfusion (SHOT) haemovigilance and progress is improving transfusion safety. *British journal of haematology.* [Review]. 2013 Nov;163(3):303-14.

[67] Matsumoto N, Akaike M, Nishiuchi T, Kawai H, Saito S. Different secretion profiles of atrial and brain natriuretic peptides after acute volume loading in patients with ischemic heart disease. *Acta Cardiol.* 1997;52(3):261-72.

[68] Watson HG, Greaves M. Can we predict bleeding? *Semin Thromb Hemost.* 2008 Feb;34(1):97-103.

[69] Puetz J. Fresh frozen plasma: the most commonly prescribed hemostatic agent. *Journal of thrombosis and haemostasis: JTH.* [Review]. 2013 Oct;11(10):1794-9.

[70] Wheeler AP, Rice TW. Coagulopathy in critically ill patients: part 2-soluble clotting factors and hemostatic testing. *Chest.* 2010 Jan;137(1):185-94.

[71] Collins PW, Macchiavello LI, Lewis SJ, Macartney NJ, Saayman AG, Luddington R, et al. Global tests of haemostasis in critically ill patients with severe sepsis syndrome compared to controls. *Br J Haematol.* 2006 Oct;135(2):220-7.

[72] Tripodi A, Primignani M, Chantarangkul V, Mannucci PM. More on: enhanced thrombin generation in patients with cirrhosis-induced coagulopathy. *J Thromb Haemost.* 2011 Mar;9(3):612-3; author reply 3-14.

[73] Chowdhury P, Saayman AG, Paulus U, Findlay GP, Collins PW. Efficacy of standard dose and 30 ml/kg fresh frozen plasma in correcting laboratory parameters of haemostasis in critically ill patients. *Br J Haematol*. 2004 Apr;125(1):69-73.

[74] McVay PA, Toy PT. Lack of increased bleeding after paracentesis and thoracentesis in patients with mild coagulation abnormalities. *Transfusion*. 1991 Feb;31(2):164-71.

[75] McVay PA, Toy PT. Lack of increased bleeding after liver biopsy in patients with mild hemostatic abnormalities. *Am J Clin Pathol*. 1990 Dec;94(6):747-53.

[76] Ng VL. Liver disease, coagulation testing, and hemostasis. *Clin Lab Med*. 2009 Jun;29(2):265-82.

[77] Trotter JF, Olson J, Lefkowitz J, Smith AD, Arjal R, Kenison J. Changes in international normalized ratio (INR) and model for endstage liver disease (MELD) based on selection of clinical laboratory. American journal of transplantation: official journal of the American Society of Transplantation and the American Society of Transplant Surgeons. [Multicenter Study]. 2007 Jun;7(6):1624-8.

[78] Porte RJ, Lisman T, Tripodi A, Caldwell SH, Trotter JF. The International Normalized Ratio (INR) in the MELD score: problems and solutions. *Am J Transplant. 2010* Jun;10(6):1349-53.

[79] El-Jack SS, Ruygrok PN, Webster MW, Stewart JT, Bass NM, Armstrong GP, et al. Effectiveness of manual pressure hemostasis following transfemoral coronary angiography in patients on therapeutic warfarin anticoagulation. *Am J Cardiol*. 2006 Feb 15;97(4):485-8.

[80] Ihezue CU, Smart J, Dewbury KC, Mehta R, Burgess L. Biopsy of the prostate guided by transrectal ultrasound: relation between warfarin use and incidence of bleeding complications. *Clin Radiol*. 2005 Apr;60(4):459-63; discussion 7-8.

[81] Grobler C, Callum J, McCluskey SA. Reversal of vitamin K antagonists prior to urgent surgery. *Can J Anaesth*. 2010 May;57(5):458-67.

[82] Sarode R, Rawal A, Lee R, Shen YM, Frenkel EP. Poor correlation of supratherapeutic international normalised ratio and vitamin K-dependent procoagulant factor levels during warfarin therapy. *Br J Haematol*. 2006 Mar;132(5):604-7.

[83] Matevosyan K, Madden C, Barnett SL, Beshay JE, Rutherford C, Sarode R. Coagulation factor levels in neurosurgical patients with mild prolongation of prothrombin time: effect on plasma transfusion therapy. *J Neurosurg*. 2011 Jan;114(1):3-7.

[84] Gulati G, Hevelow M, George M, Behling E, Siegel J. International normalized ratio versus plasma levels of coagulation factors in patients on vitamin K antagonist therapy. *Arch Pathol Lab Med.* 2011 Apr;135(4):490-4.

[85] Lind SE, Callas PW, Golden EA, Joyner KA, Jr., Ortel TL. Plasma levels of factors II, VII and X and their relationship to the international normalized ratio during chronic warfarin therapy. *Blood Coagul Fibrinolysis.* 1997 Jan;8(1):48-53.

[86] Loewen P, Dahri K. Risk of bleeding with oral anticoagulants: an updated systematic review and performance analysis of clinical prediction rules. *Ann Hematol.* 2011 Oct;90(10):1191-200.

[87] Segal JB, Dzik WH. Paucity of studies to support that abnormal coagulation test results predict bleeding in the setting of invasive procedures: an evidence-based review. *Transfusion.* 2005 Sep;45(9):1413-25.

[88] Chee YL, Crawford JC, Watson HG, Greaves M. Guidelines on the assessment of bleeding risk prior to surgery or invasive procedures. British Committee for Standards in Haematology. *Br J Haematol.* 2008 Mar;140(5):496-504.

[89] Eckman MH, Erban JK, Singh SK, Kao GS. Screening for the risk for bleeding or thrombosis. *Ann Intern Med.* 2003 Feb 4;138(3):W15-24.

[90] Makris M, Greaves M, Phillips WS, Kitchen S, Rosendaal FR, Preston EF. Emergency oral anticoagulant reversal: the relative efficacy of infusions of fresh frozen plasma and clotting factor concentrate on correction of the coagulopathy. *Thromb Haemost.* 1997 Mar;77(3):477-80.

[91] Burns ER, Goldberg SN, Wenz B. Paradoxic effect of multiple mild coagulation factor deficiencies on the prothrombin time and activated partial thromboplastin time. *American journal of clinical pathology.* 1993 Aug;100(2):94-8.

[92] Tripodi A, Primignani M, Chantarangkul V, Dell'Era A, Clerici M, de Franchis R, et al. An imbalance of pro- vs. anti-coagulation factors in plasma from patients with cirrhosis. *Gastroenterology.* 2009 Dec;137(6):2105-11.

[93] Deitcher SR. Interpretation of the international normalised ratio in patients with liver disease. *Lancet.* 2002 Jan 5;359(9300):47-8.

[94] Mannucci PM, Franchi F, Dioguardi N. Correction of abnormal coagulation in chronic liver disease by combined use of fresh-frozen

plasma and prothrombin complex concentrates. *Lancet.* 1976 Sep 11;2(7985):542-5.

[95] Kovacs MJ, Wong A, MacKinnon K, Weir K, Keeney M, Boyle E, et al. Assessment of the validity of the INR system for patients with liver impairment. *Thromb Haemost.* 1994 Jun;71(6):727-30.

[96] Levy JH, Dutton RP, Hemphill JC, 3rd, Shander A, Cooper D, Paidas MJ, et al. Multidisciplinary approach to the challenge of hemostasis. *Anesth Analg.* 2010 Feb 1;110(2):354-64.

[97] Levi M, van der Poll T. Inflammation and coagulation. *Crit Care Med.* 2010 Feb;38(2 Suppl):S26-34.

[98] Hoffman M, Monroe DM, 3rd. A cell-based model of hemostasis. *Thrombosis and haemostasis.* [Review]. 2001 Jun;85(6):958-65.

[99] Tripodi A, Mannucci PM. The coagulopathy of chronic liver disease. *N Engl J Med.* 2011 Jul 14;365(2):147-56.

[100] Northup PG. Hypercoagulation in liver disease. *Clin Liver Dis.* 2009 Feb;13(1):109-16.

[101] Senzolo M, Sartori MT, Lisman T. Should we give thromboprophylaxis to patients with liver cirrhosis and coagulopathy? HPB (Oxford). 2009 Sep;11(6):459-64.

[102] Abdel-Wahab OI, Healy B, Dzik WH. Effect of fresh-frozen plasma transfusion on prothrombin time and bleeding in patients with mild coagulation abnormalities. *Transfusion.* 2006 Aug;46(8):1279-85.

[103] Youssef WI, Salazar F, Dasarathy S, Beddow T, Mullen KD. Role of fresh frozen plasma infusion in correction of coagulopathy of chronic liver disease: a dual phase study. *Am J Gastroenterol.* 2003 Jun;98(6):1391-4.

[104] Spector I, Corn M, Ticktin HE. Effect of plasma transfusions on the prothrombin time and clotting factors in liver disease. *N Engl J Med.* 1966 Nov 10;275(19):1032-7.

[105] Tinmouth A. Evidence for a rationale use of frozen plasma for the treatment and prevention of bleeding. Transfusion and apheresis science: official journal of the World Apheresis Association: *official journal of the European Society for Haemapheresis.* [Research Support, Non-U.S. Gov't Review]. 2012 Jun;46(3):293-8.

[106] Holland LL, Foster TM, Marlar RA, Brooks JP. Fresh frozen plasma is ineffective for correcting minimally elevated international normalized ratios. *Transfusion.* 2005 Jul;45(7):1234-5.

[107] Shinagare SA, Angarkar NN, Desai SR, Naniwadekar MR. An audit of fresh frozen plasma usage and effect of fresh frozen plasma on the pre-

transfusion international normalized ratio. *Asian J Transfus Sci.* 2010 Jul;4(2):128-32.

[108] Gray OP, Ackerman A, Fraser AJ. Intracranial haemorrhage and clotting defects in low-birth-weight infants. *Lancet.* 1968 Mar 16;1(7542):545-8.

[109] Gazzard BG, Henderson JM, Williams R. The use of fresh frozen plasma or a concentrate of factor IX as replacement therapy before liver biopsy. *Gut.* 1975 Aug;16(8):621-5.

[110] Muller MC, Straat M, Meijers JC, Klinkspoor JH, de Jonge E, Arbous MS, et al. Fresh frozen plasma transfusion fails to influence the hemostatic balance in critically ill patients with a coagulopathy. *J Thromb Haemost.* 2015 Mar 21.

[111] Murad MH, Stubbs JR, Gandhi MJ, Wang AT, Paul A, Erwin PJ, et al. The effect of plasma transfusion on morbidity and mortality: a systematic review and meta-analysis. *Transfusion.* 2010 Jun;50(6):1370-83.

[112] Desborough MJ, Stanworth SJ. Uses and abuses of fresh-frozen plasma for the prophylaxis of bleeding. *Clin Med.* 2013 Apr;13(2):197-9.

[113] Muller MC, de Haan RJ, Vroom MB, Juffermans NP. Evaluation of a multi-center randomised clinical trial on prophylactic transfusion of fresh frozen plasma: implications for future trials. *Transfusion medicine.* 2014 Oct;24(5):292-6.

[114] Karam O, Tucci M, Combescure C, Lacroix J, Rimensberger PC. Plasma transfusion strategies for critically ill patients. *Cochrane Database Syst Rev.* 2013;12:CD010654.

[115] Jansen TC, Kompanje EJ, Bakker J. Deferred proxy consent in emergency critical care research: ethically valid and practically feasible. *Critical care medicine.* 2009 Jan;37(1 Suppl):S65-8.

[116] Veelo DP, Vlaar AP, Dongelmans DA, Binnekade JM, Levi M, Paulus F, et al. Correction of subclinical coagulation disorders before percutaneous dilatational tracheotomy. *Blood transfusion = Trasfusione del sangue. [Randomized Controlled Trial].* 2012 Apr;10(2):213-20.

[117] Barnette RE, Fish DJ, Eisenstaedt RS. Modification of fresh-frozen plasma transfusion practices through educational intervention. *Transfusion.* 1990 Mar-Apr;30(3):253-7.

[118] Damiani G, Pinnarelli L, Sommella L, Farelli V, Mele L, Menichella G, et al. Appropriateness of fresh-frozen plasma usage in hospital settings: a meta-analysis of the impact of organizational interventions. *Transfusion.* 2010 Jan;50(1):139-44.

[119] Kakkar N, Kaur R, Dhanoa J. Improvement in fresh frozen plasma transfusion practice: results of an outcome audit. *Transfus Med.* 2004 Jun;14(3):231-5.

[120] Shanberge JN. Reduction of fresh-frozen plasma use through a daily survey and education program. *Transfusion.* 1987 May-Jun;27(3):226-7.

[121] Tavares M, DiQuattro P, Nolette N, Conti G, Sweeney J. Reduction in plasma transfusion after enforcement of transfusion guidelines. *Transfusion.* 2011 Apr;51(4):754-61.

[122] Tuckfield A, Haeusler MN, Grigg AP, Metz J. Reduction of inappropriate use of blood products by prospective monitoring of transfusion request forms. *Med J Aust.* 1997 Nov 3;167(9):473-6.

[123] Pendergrast J. Urgent warfarin reversal: know your options. *Can J Anaesth.* 2010 May;57(5):395-401.

[124] Bonhomme F, Ajzenberg N, Schved JF, Molliex S, Samama CM. Pre-interventional haemostatic assessment: Guidelines from the French Society of Anaesthesia and Intensive Care. *European journal of anaesthesiology.* [Research Support, Non-U.S. Gov't]. 2013 Apr;30(4):142-62.

[125] Johansson PI, Stissing T, Bochsen L, Ostrowski SR. Thrombelastography and tromboelastometry in assessing coagulopathy in trauma. *Scand J Trauma Resusc Emerg Med.* 2009;17:45.

[126] Perry DJ, Fitzmaurice DA, Kitchen S, Mackie IJ, Mallett S. Point-of-care testing in haemostasis. *British journal of haematology.* [Review]. 2010 Sep;150(5):501-14.

[127] Ganter MT, Hofer CK. Coagulation monitoring: current techniques and clinical use of viscoelastic point-of-care coagulation devices. *Anesth Analg.* 2008 May;106(5):1366-75.

[128] Coakley M, Reddy K, Mackie I, Mallett S. Transfusion triggers in orthotopic liver transplantation: a comparison of the thromboelastometry analyzer, the thromboelastogram, and conventional coagulation tests. *J Cardiothorac Vasc Anesth.* 2006 Aug;20(4):548-53.

[129] Trzebicki J, Flakiewicz E, Kosieradzki M, Blaszczyk B, Kolacz M, Jureczko L, et al. The use of thromboelastometry in the assessment of hemostasis during orthotopic liver transplantation reduces the demand for blood products. *Ann Transplant.* 2010 Sep 28;15(3):19-24.

[130] Ronald A, Dunning J. Can the use of thromboelastography predict and decrease bleeding and blood and blood product requirements in adult patients undergoing cardiac surgery? *Interact Cardiovasc Thorac Surg.* 2005 Oct;4(5):456-63.

[131] Dunning J, Versteegh M, Fabbri A, Pavie A, Kolh P, Lockowandt U, et al. Guideline on antiplatelet and anticoagulation management in cardiac surgery. *Eur J Cardiothorac Surg*. 2008 Jul;34(1):73-92.

[132] Gorlinger K, Dirkmann D, Hanke AA. Potential value of transfusion protocols in cardiac surgery. *Current opinion in anaesthesiology*. [Review]. 2013 Apr;26(2):230-43.

[133] Schochl H, Nienaber U, Hofer G, Voelckel W, Jambor C, Scharbert G, et al. Goal-directed coagulation management of major trauma patients using thromboelastometry (ROTEM)-guided administration of fibrinogen concentrate and prothrombin complex concentrate. *Critical care*. 2010;14(2):R55.

[134] Holcomb JB, Minei KM, Scerbo ML, Radwan ZA, Wade CE, Kozar RA, et al. Admission rapid thrombelastography can replace conventional coagulation tests in the emergency department: experience with 1974 consecutive trauma patients. *Annals of surgery*. [Comparative Study Evaluation Studies Research Support, Non-U.S. Gov't Research Support, U.S. Gov't, Non-P.H.S.]. 2012 Sep;256(3):476-86.

[135] de Lange NM, Lance MD, de Groot R, Beckers EA, Henskens YM, Scheepers HC. Obstetric hemorrhage and coagulation: an update. Thromboelastography, thromboelastometry, and conventional coagulation tests in the diagnosis and prediction of postpartum hemorrhage. *Obstet Gynecol Surv*. [Review]. 2012 Jul;67(7):426-35.

[136] Al Hawaj MA, Martin EJ, Venitz J, Barrett JC, Kuhn JG, Nolte ME, et al. Monitoring rFVIII prophylaxis dosing using global haemostasis assays. *Haemophilia*. 2013 May;19(3):409-14.

[137] Chitlur M, Warrier I, Rajpurkar M, Hollon W, Llanto L, Wiseman C, et al. Thromboelastography in children with coagulation factor deficiencies. *Br J Haematol*. 2008 Jun;142(2):250-6.

[138] Zia AN, Chitlur M, Rajpurkar M, Ozgonenel B, Lusher J, Callaghan JH, et al. Thromboelastography identifies children with rare bleeding disorders and predicts bleeding phenotype. *Haemophilia*. 2015 Jan;21(1):124-32.

[139] Schochl H, Nienaber U, Hofer G, Voelckel W, Jambor C, Scharbert G, et al. Goal-directed coagulation management of major trauma patients using thromboelastometry (ROTEM)-guided administration of fibrinogen concentrate and prothrombin complex concentrate. *Crit Care*. 2010;14(2):R55.

[140] Hunt H, Stanworth S, Curry N, Woolley T, Cooper C, Ukoumunne O, et al. Thromboelastography (TEG) and rotational thromboelastometry

(ROTEM) for traumainduced coagulopathy in adult trauma patients with bleeding. *Cochrane Database Syst Rev*. 2015 Feb 16;2:CD010438.

[141] Gurusamy KS, Pissanou T, Pikhart H, Vaughan J, Burroughs AK, Davidson BR. Methods to decrease blood loss and transfusion requirements for liver transplantation. *The Cochrane database of systematic reviews*. [Meta-Analysis Review]. 2011(12):CD009052.

[142] Wang SC, Shieh JF, Chang KY, Chu YC, Liu CS, Loong CC, et al. Thromboelastography-guided transfusion decreases intraoperative blood transfusion during orthotopic liver transplantation: randomized clinical trial. *Transplantation proceedings*. [Randomized Controlled Trial Research Support, Non-U.S. Gov't]. 2010 Sep;42(7):2590-3.

[143] L. De Pietri MB, R. Montalti, T. Di Maira, N. De Maria, B. Begliomini, G.E. Gerunda, E. Villa. Thrombelastography before invasive procedures reduces hemoderivates requirement in cirrhotic patients with coagulation disorders. A randomized controlled trial. *Journal of Hepatology* -. April 2013 (Vol. 58Supplement 1, Pages S85-S86, DOI: 10.1016/S0168-8278(13)60196-8).

[144] Tripodi A, Salerno F, Chantarangkul V, Clerici M, Cazzaniga M, Primignani M, et al. Evidence of normal thrombin generation in cirrhosis despite abnormal conventional coagulation tests. *Hepatology*. 2005 Mar;41(3):553-8.

[145] Mallett SV, Chowdary P, Burroughs AK. Clinical utility of viscoelastic tests of coagulation in patients with liver disease. *Liver international: official journal of the International Association for the Study of the Liver*. 2013 Aug;33(7):961-74.

[146] Dupont J, Messiant F, Declerck N, Tavernier B, Jude B, Durinck L, et al. Liver transplantation without the use of fresh frozen plasma. *Anesth Analg*. 1996 Oct;83(4):681-6.

[147] Kozek-Langenecker SA, Afshari A, Albaladejo P, Santullano CA, De Robertis E, Filipescu DC, et al. Management of severe perioperative bleeding: Guidelines from the European Society of Anaesthesiology. *European journal of anaesthesiology*. 2013 Jun;30(6):270-382.

[148] Madsen DE, Ingerslev J, Sidelmann JJ, Thorn JJ, Gram J. Intraoperative blood loss during orthognathic surgery is predicted by thromboelastography. *J Oral Maxillofac Surg*. [Comparative Study]. 2012 Oct;70(10):e547-52.

[149] Butwick A, Ting V, Ralls LA, Harter S, Riley E. The association between thromboelastographic parameters and total estimated blood loss in patients undergoing elective cesarean delivery. *Anesthesia and*

analgesia. [Research Support, Non-U.S. Gov't]. 2011 May;112(5):1041-7.

[150] Davis CL, Chandler WL. Thromboelastography for the prediction of bleeding after transplant renal biopsy. *J Am Soc Nephrol.* 1995 Oct;6(4):1250-5.

[151] Souto LR, Chaim EA, Barbosa RC, Bizzacchi JM. Increased intraoperative bleeding in patients undergoing abdominoplasty after gastroplasty is not due to coagulopathy. *Aesthetic Plast Surg.* [Research Support, Non-U.S. Gov't]. 2012 Dec;36(6):1283-91.

[152] El Kady N, Khedr H, Yosry M, El Mekawi S. Perioperative assessment of coagulation in paediatric neurosurgical patients using thromboelastography. *European journal of anaesthesiology.* [Evaluation Studies]. 2009 Apr;26(4):293-7.

[153] Vieira da Rocha EC, D'Amico EA, Caldwell SH, Flores da Rocha TR, Soares ESCS, Dos Santos Bomfim V, et al. A prospective study of conventional and expanded coagulation indices in predicting ulcer bleeding after variceal band ligation. *Clin Gastroenterol Hepatol.* 2009 Sep;7(9):988-93.

[154] Park MS, Martini WZ, Dubick MA, Salinas J, Butenas S, Kheirabadi BS, et al. Thromboelastography as a better indicator of hypercoagulable state after injury than prothrombin time or activated partial thromboplastin time. *J Trauma.* 2009 Aug;67(2):266-75; discussion 75-6.

[155] Rugeri L, Levrat A, David JS, Delecroix E, Floccard B, Gros A, et al. Diagnosis of early coagulation abnormalities in trauma patients by rotation thrombelastography. *J Thromb Haemost.* 2007 Feb;5(2):289-95.

[156] Agren A, Wikman AT, Holmstrom M, Ostlund A, Edgren G. Thromboelastography (TEG(R)) compared to conventional coagulation tests in surgical patients--a laboratory evaluation. *Scand J Clin Lab Invest.* 2013 Apr;73(3):214-20.

[157] Nascimento B, Al Mahoos M, Callum J, Capone A, Pacher J, Tien H, et al. Vitamin K-dependent coagulation factor deficiency in trauma: a comparative analysis between international normalized ratio and thromboelastography. *Transfusion.* 2011 Jul 11.

[158] Hepner DL, Concepcion M, Bhavani-Shankar K. Coagulation status using thromboelastography in patients receiving warfarin prophylaxis and epidural analgesia. *J Clin Anesth.* 2002 Sep;14(6):405-10.

[159] Fries D, Haas T, Klingler A, Streif W, Klima G, Martini J, et al. Efficacy of fibrinogen and prothrombin complex concentrate used to reverse

dilutional coagulopathy--a porcine model. *Br J Anaesth.* 2006 Oct;97(4):460-7.

[160] Venema LF, Post WJ, Hendriks HG, Huet RC, de Wolf JT, de Vries AJ. An assessment of clinical interchangeability of TEG and RoTEM thromboelastographic variables in cardiac surgical patients. *Anesthesia and analgesia.* [Comparative Study]. 2010 Aug;111(2):339-44.

[161] Sankarankutty A, Nascimento B, Teodoro da Luz L, Rizoli S. TEG(R) and ROTEM(R) in trauma: similar test but different results? *World J Emerg Surg.* 2012 Aug 22;7 Suppl 1:S3.

[162] Muller MC, Meijers JC, Vroom MB, Juffermans NP. Utility of thromboelastography and/or thromboelastometry in adults with sepsis: a systematic review. *Crit Care.* 2014;18(1):R30.

[163] Mannucci PM. Abnormal hemostasis tests and bleeding in chronic liver disease: are they related? *No. J Thromb Haemost.* 2006 Apr;4(4):721-3.

[164] Massicotte L, Beaulieu D, Thibeault L, Roy JD, Marleau D, Lapointe R, et al. Coagulation defects do not predict blood product requirements during liver transplantation. Transplantation. 2008 Apr 15;85(7):956-62.

[165] Ewe K. Bleeding after liver biopsy does not correlate with indices of peripheral coagulation. *Digestive diseases and sciences.* 1981 May;26(5):388-93.

[166] Gilmore IT, Burroughs A, Murray-Lyon IM, Williams R, Jenkins D, Hopkins A. Indications, methods, and outcomes of percutaneous liver biopsy in England and Wales: an audit by the British Society of Gastroenterology and the Royal College of Physicians of London. *Gut.* 1995 Mar;36(3):437-41.

[167] McGill DB, Rakela J, Zinsmeister AR, Ott BJ. A 21-year experience with major hemorrhage after percutaneous liver biopsy. *Gastroenterology.* 1990 Nov;99(5):1396-400.

[168] Caturelli E, Squillante MM, Andriulli A, Siena DA, Cellerino C, De Luca F, et al. Fine-needle liver biopsy in patients with severely impaired coagulation. *Liver.* 1993 Oct;13(5):270-3.

[169] Matsumoto M, Kawa K, Uemura M, Kato S, Ishizashi H, Isonishi A, et al. Prophylactic fresh frozen plasma may prevent development of hepatic VOD after stem cell transplantation via ADAMTS13-mediated restoration of von Willebrand factor plasma levels. *Bone marrow transplantation.* [Multicenter Study Randomized Controlled Trial Research Support, Non-U.S. Gov't]. 2007 Aug;40(3):251-9.

[170] Massicotte L, Lenis S, Thibeault L, Sassine MP, Seal RF, Roy A. Reduction of blood product transfusions during liver transplantation. *Can J Anaesth*. 2005 May;52(5):545-6.

[171] Massicotte L, Lenis S, Thibeault L, Sassine MP, Seal RF, Roy A. Effect of low central venous pressure and phlebotomy on blood product transfusion requirements during liver transplantations. *Liver Transpl.* 2006 Jan;12(1):117-23.

[172] Lisman T, Caldwell SH, Burroughs AK, Northup PG, Senzolo M, Stravitz RT, et al. Hemostasis and thrombosis in patients with liver disease: the ups and downs. *J Hepatol.* 2010 Aug;53(2):362-71.

[173] Gatt A, Riddell A, Calvaruso V, Tuddenham EG, Makris M, Burroughs AK. Enhanced thrombin generation in patients with cirrhosis-induced coagulopathy. *J Thromb Haemost*. 2010 Sep;8(9):1994-2000.

[174] Munoz SJ, Stravitz RT, Gabriel DA. Coagulopathy of acute liver failure. *Clin Liver Dis.* 2009 Feb;13(1):95-107.

[175] Stravitz RT, Lisman T, Luketic VA, Sterling RK, Puri P, Fuchs M, et al. Minimal effects of acute liver injury/acute liver failure on hemostasis as assessed by thromboelastography. *J Hepatol.* 2011 May 19.

[176] Gazzard BG, Henderson JM, Williams R. Early changes in coagulation following a paracetamol overdose and a controlled trial of fresh frozen plasma therapy. *Gut.* [Clinical Trial Randomized Controlled Trial]. 1975 Aug;16(8):617-20.

[177] Vaquero J, Fontana RJ, Larson AM, Bass NM, Davern TJ, Shakil AO, et al. Complications and use of intracranial pressure monitoring in patients with acute liver failure and severe encephalopathy. *Liver Transpl.* 2005 Dec;11(12):1581-9.

[178] Le TV, Rumbak MJ, Liu SS, Alsina AE, van Loveren H, Agazzi S. Insertion of intracranial pressure monitors in fulminant hepatic failure patients: early experience using recombinant factor VII. *Neurosurgery.* 2010 Mar;66(3):455-8; discussion 8.

[179] Shami VM, Caldwell SH, Hespenheide EE, Arseneau KO, Bickston SJ, Macik BG. Recombinant activated factor VII for coagulopathy in fulminant hepatic failure compared with conventional therapy. *Liver Transpl.* 2003 Feb;9(2):138-43.

[180] Lorenz R, Kienast J, Otto U, Egger K, Kiehl M, Schreiter D, et al. Efficacy and safety of a prothrombin complex concentrate with two virus-inactivation steps in patients with severe liver damage. *Eur J Gastroenterol Hepatol.* 2003 Jan;15(1):15-20.

[181] Blonski W, Siropaides T, Reddy KR. Coagulopathy in liver disease. *Curr Treat Options Gastroenterol.* 2007 Dec;10(6):464-73.
[182] Stravitz RT. Critical management decisions in patients with acute liver failure. *Chest.* 2008 Nov;134(5):1092-102.
[183] Mumtaz H, Williams V, Hauer-Jensen M, Rowe M, Henry-Tillman RS, Heaton K, et al. Central venous catheter placement in patients with disorders of hemostasis. *Am J Surg.* 2000 Dec;180(6):503-5; discussion 6.
[184] Haas B, Chittams JL, Trerotola SO. Large-bore tunneled central venous catheter insertion in patients with coagulopathy. *J Vasc Interv Radiol.* 2010 Feb;21(2):212-7.
[185] Weigand K, Encke J, Meyer FJ, Hinkel UP, Munder M, Stremmel W, et al. Low levels of prothrombin time (INR) and platelets do not increase the risk of significant bleeding when placing central venous catheters. *Med Klin* (Munich). 2009 May 15;104(5):331-5.
[186] Carino GP, Tsapenko AV, Sweeney JD. Central line placement in patients with and without prophylactic plasma. *J Crit Care.* 2012 Oct;27(5):529 e9-13.
[187] Della Vigna P, Monfardini L, Bonomo G, Curigliano G, Agazzi A, Bellomi M, et al. Coagulation disorders in patients with cancer: nontunneled central venous catheter placement with US guidance--a single-institution retrospective analysis. *Radiology.* 2009 Oct;253(1):249-52.
[188] Doerfler ME, Kaufman B, Goldenberg AS. Central venous catheter placement in patients with disorders of hemostasis. *Chest.* 1996 Jul;110(1):185-8.
[189] DeLoughery TG, Liebler JM, Simonds V, Goodnight SH. Invasive line placement in critically ill patients: do hemostatic defects matter? *Transfusion.* 1996 Sep;36(9):827-31.
[190] Putensen C, Theuerkauf N, Guenther U, Vargas M, Pelosi P. Percutaneous and surgical tracheostomy in critically ill adult patients: a meta-analysis. *Crit Care.* 2014 Dec 19;18(6):544.
[191] Sanabria A. Which percutaneous tracheostomy method is better? A systematic review. *Respir Care.* 2014 Nov;59(11):1660-70.
[192] Bass J, White DA. Thoracentesis in patients with hematologic malignancy: yield and safety. *Chest.* 2005 Jun;127(6):2101-5.
[193] Hibbert RM, Atwell TD, Lekah A, Patel MD, Carter RE, McDonald JS, et al. Safety of ultrasound-guided thoracentesis in patients with abnormal preprocedural coagulation parameters. *Chest.* 2013 Aug;144(2):456-63.

[194] Patel MD, Joshi SD. Abnormal preprocedural international normalized ratio and platelet counts are not associated with increased bleeding complications after ultrasound-guided thoracentesis. *AJR Am J Roentgenol.* 2011 Jul;197(1):W164-8.
[195] Puchalski JT, Argento AC, Murphy TE, Araujo KL, Pisani MA. The safety of thoracentesis in patients with uncorrected bleeding risk. *Ann Am Thorac Soc.* 2013 Aug;10(4):336-41.
[196] Puchalski J. Thoracentesis and the risks for bleeding: a new era. *Curr Opin Pulm Med.* 2014 Jul;20(4):377-84.
[197] McCall MM, Blackwell MM, Smyre JT, Sistino JJ, Acsell JR, Dorman BH, et al. Fresh frozen plasma in the pediatric pump prime: a prospective, randomized trial. *The Annals of thoracic surgery.* [Clinical Trial Randomized Controlled Trial]. 2004 Mar;77(3):983-7; discussion 7.
[198] Boldt J, von Bormann B, Kling D, Jacobi M, Moosdorf R, Hempelmann G. Preoperative plasmapheresis in patients undergoing cardiac surgery procedures. *Anesthesiology.* [Clinical Trial Randomized Controlled Trial]. 1990 Feb;72(2):282-8.
[199] Boldt J, Zickmann B, Ballesteros M, Oehmke S, Stertmann F, Hempelmann G. Influence of acute preoperative plasmapheresis on platelet function in cardiac surgery. *Journal of cardiothoracic and vascular anesthesia.* [Clinical Trial Controlled Clinical Trial Randomized Controlled Trial]. 1993 Feb;7(1):4-9.
[200] Menges T, Welters I, Wagner RM, Boldt J, Dapper F, Hempelmann G. The influence of acute preoperative plasmapheresis on coagulation tests, fibrinolysis, blood loss and transfusion requirements in cardiac surgery. European journal of cardio-thoracic surgery: *official journal of the European Association for Cardio-thoracic Surgery.* [Clinical Trial Randomized Controlled Trial]. 1997 Mar;11(3):557-63.
[201] Casbard AC, Williamson LM, Murphy MF, Rege K, Johnson T. The role of prophylactic fresh frozen plasma in decreasing blood loss and correcting coagulopathy in cardiac surgery. A systematic review. *Anaesthesia.* [Meta-Analysis Research Support, Non-U.S. Gov't Review]. 2004 Jun;59(6):550-8.
[202] Aad G, Abajyan T, Abbott B, Abdallah J, Abdel Khalek S, Abdelalim AA, et al. Observation of Associated Near-Side and Away-Side Long-Range Correlations in sqrt[s_{NN}]=5.02 TeV Proton-Lead Collisions with the ATLAS Detector. Phys Rev Lett. 2013 May 3;110(18):182302.

[203] Davis JW, Davis IC, Bennink LD, Hysell SE, Curtis BV, Kaups KL, et al. Placement of intracranial pressure monitors: are "normal" coagulation parameters necessary? *The Journal of trauma*. 2004 Dec;57(6):1173-7.

[204] Gerlach R, Krause M, Seifert V, Goerlinger K. Hemostatic and hemorrhagic problems in neurosurgical patients. *Acta Neurochir* (Wien). 2009 Aug;151(8):873-900; discussion

[205] Beshay JE, Morgan H, Madden C, Yu W, Sarode R. Emergency reversal of anticoagulation and antiplatelet therapies in neurosurgical patients. *J Neurosurg*. 2010 Feb;112(2):307-18.

[206] Etemadrezaie H, Baharvahdat H, Shariati Z, Lari SM, Shakeri MT, Ganjeifar B. The effect of fresh frozen plasma in severe closed head injury. *Clin Neurol Neurosurg*. 2007 Feb;109(2):166-71.

[207] Schramm B, Leslie K, Myles PS, Hogan CJ. Coagulation studies in preoperative neurosurgical patients. *Anaesthesia and intensive care*. 2001 Aug;29(4):388-92.

[208] Keeling D, Baglin T, Tait C, Watson H, Perry D, Baglin C, et al. Guidelines on oral anticoagulation with warfarin - fourth edition. *British journal of haematology*. [Practice Guideline Review]. 2011 Aug;154(3):311-24.

[209] Yiu KH, Siu CW, Jim MH, Tse HF, Fan K, Chau MC, et al. Comparison of the efficacy and safety profiles of intravenous vitamin K and fresh frozen plasma as treatment of warfarin-related over-anticoagulation in patients with mechanical heart valves. *Am J Cardiol*. 2006 Feb 1;97(3):409-11.

[210] Demeyere R, Gillardin S, Arnout J, Strengers PF. Comparison of fresh frozen plasma and prothrombin complex concentrate for the reversal of oral anticoagulants in patients undergoing cardiopulmonary bypass surgery: a randomized study. *Vox Sang*. 2010 Oct;99(3):251-60.

[211] Stanworth SJ, Brunskill SJ, Hyde CJ, McClelland DB, Murphy MF. Is fresh frozen plasma clinically effective? A systematic review of randomized controlled trials. *Br J Haematol*. 2004 Jul;126(1):139-52.

[212] Streiff MB. Prothrombin complex concentrates for reversal of vitamin K antagonists: assessing the risks. *Thromb Haemost*. 2011 Sep;106(3):389-90.

[213] Schochl H, Voelckel W, Maegele M, Kirchmair L, Schlimp CJ. Endogenous thrombin potential following hemostatic therapy with 4-factor prothrombin complex concentrate: a 7-day observational study of trauma patients. *Critical care*. [Research Support, Non-U.S. Gov't]. 2014;18(4):R147.

Mannucci PM, Franchini M. Recombinant factor VIIa as haemostatic therapy in advanced liver disease. *Blood transfusion* = Trasfusione del sangue. [Review]. 2013 Oct;11(4):487-90.

Index

B

C

D

E

F

G

H

I

J

K

L

M

N

O

P

Q

R

S

T

U

V

W

X

Z